International Perspectives on Public Health and Palliative Ca

Public health approaches to palliative care have been growing in policy importance and practice acceptance. This innovative volume explores the major concepts, practice examples, and practice guidelines for this new approach.

The goal of 'comprehensive care' – seamless support for patients as they transition between home-based care and inpatient services – relies on the principles of health promotion and community development to ensure services are both available and importantly appropriate for patients' needs. In developing contexts, where hospitals and hospices may be inaccessible, a public health approach provides not only continuity of care but greater access to good end of life care. This book provides both an historical and conceptual overview whilst offering practical case examples from affluent and developing contexts, in a range of clinical settings. Finally, it draws together research-based guidelines for future practice.

Essential reading for public health researchers and practitioners with an interest in end of life care and global health as well as those involved in developing palliative care provision, *International Perspectives on Public Health and Palliative Care* is the first volume to present an overview of theory and practice in this emerging field.

Libby Sallnow is a palliative medicine registrar at St Joseph's Hospice, London and is the Research Associate at the WHO Collaborating Centre for Community Participation in Palliative Care and Long Term Care, Kerala.

Suresh Kumar is currently the Director of the WHO Collaborating Centre for Community Participation in Palliative Care and Long Term Care.

Allan Kellehear is Professor, School of Health Administration, Dalhousie University, Halifax, Nova Scotia, Canada. He was formerly the Professor of Palliative Care at La Trobe University and was director of Australia's first policy and practice palliative care unit in a school of public health.

Routledge Studies in Public Health

Available titles include:

Planning in Health Promotion Work
Roar Amdam

Alcohol, Tobacco and Obesity
Morality, mortality and the new public health
Edited by Kirsten Bell, Amy Salmon and Darlene McNaughton

Population Mental Health
Evidence, policy, and public health practice
Edited by Neal Cohen and Sandro Galea

International Perspectives on Public Health and Palliative Care
Edited by Libby Sallnow, Suresh Kumar and Allan Kellehear

International Perspectives on Public Health and Palliative Care

Edited by Libby Sallnow, Suresh Kumar and Allan Kellehear

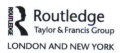
Routledge
Taylor & Francis Group

LONDON AND NEW YORK

First published 2012
by Routledge
2 Park Square, Milton Park, Abingdon, Oxon OX14 4RN

Simultaneously published in the USA and Canada
by Routledge
711 Third Avenue, New York, NY 10017 (8th Floor)

Routledge is an imprint of the Taylor & Francis Group, an informa business

First issued in paperback 2013

British Library Cataloguing in Publication Data
A catalogue record for this book is available from the British Library

Library of Congress Cataloging in Publication Data
International perspectives on public health and palliative care / edited by
Libby Sallnow, Suresh Kumar, and Allan Kellehear.
 p. ; cm. – (Routledge studies in public health)
 Includes bibliographical references.
 1. Palliative treatment. 2. Public health–International cooperation. I.
Sallnow, Libby. II. Kumar, Suresh, 1961- III. Kellehear, Allan, 1955- IV.
Series: Routledge studies in public health.
 [DNLM: 1. Palliative Care–methods. 2. Palliative Care–standards. 3.
International Cooperation. 4. Models, Organizational. 5. Public Health–
methods. 6. Public Health–standards. WB 310]
 R726.8I573 2012
 362.1–dc23

2011014007

ISBN: 978-0-415-66350-2 (hbk)
ISBN: 978-0-415-83347-9 (pbk)
ISBN: 978-0-203-80318-9 (ebk)

Typeset in Goudy
by Wearset Ltd, Boldon, Tyne and Wear

For Michael Sallnow
(1949–1990)

Contents

Illustrations

Figures

Tables

Contributors

100 Member Committee is a committee of approximately 100 organizations and individuals, with Tsutomu Hotta, CEO of Sawayaka Welfare Foundation, serving as its chairman, Japan.

Dr Steve Conway is Senior Lecturer – Research Methods, School of Health and Social Care, Teesside University, Middlesbrough, UK.

Kathleen Dansie is Project Manager for South African HOME Hospice Project; Teacher Librarian, Australia.

Dr Julia Downing is Honorary Professor of Palliative Medicine at Makerere University, Uganda, and an International Palliative Care Consultant.

Dr Patricia Granja H. is Medical doctor and lecturer/researcher at the Institute of Public Health, Pontifical University of Ecuador.

Dr Liz Gwyther is Executive Director, Hospice and Palliative Care Association of South Africa.

Nigel Hartley is Director of Supportive Care, St Christopher's Hospice London.

Professor Allan Kellehear is Professor, School of Health Administration, Dalhousie University, Halifax, Nova Scotia, Canada.

Dr Suresh Kumar is Director of the Institute of Palliative Medicine, Kerala, India, WHO Collaborating Centre for Community Participation in Palliative Care and Long Term Care.

Gerard Manion, Medal of the Order of Australia (OAM), is Director Cancer Care Program and Co-founder HOME Hospice, Australia.

Dr Helen-Anne Manion, OAM, is Palliative Care Physician and Co-founder HOME Hospice, Australia.

Peter McLoughlin is Strategic Programme Manager, Lothian NHS Board, Edinburgh, Scotland.

Prof Scott A. Murray is St Columba's Hospice Chair of Primary Palliative Care, Primary Palliative Care Research Group, The University of Edinburgh, Scotland.

Dr Faith Mwangi-Powell is Executive Director, African Palliative Care Association, Uganda.

Dr Heather Richardson is Director of Strategy at St Joseph's Hospice, London and National Clinical Head at Help the Hospices, London.

Dr John Rosenberg is Director of the Calvary Centre for Palliative Care Research in Canberra, Australia.

Dr Bruce Rumbold is Director of the Palliative Care Unit in the School of Public Health, La Trobe University, Victoria, Australia.

Dr Libby Sallnow is a palliative medicine registrar at St Joseph's Hospice, London and research associate, WHO Collaborating Centre for Community Participation in Palliative Care and Long Term Care, Kerala.

Preface

Over the past 40 years, palliative care has made great strides in improving care for those with life-limiting diseases. A combination of international associations, reforms to opiate prescribing laws, active research and education programmes, and government strategy and policy have combined to render palliative care an accepted part of mainstream health care in many countries. However, notwithstanding these achievements, palliative care still has a long way to go. In order to solve the urgent issues of access and equity which confront low- and middle-income countries, and to address meaningful solutions to 'whole person care' of a dying person and their family, we must move beyond the bedside. In order to achieve meaningful coverage by services which truly address both symptom needs and the social, spiritual and psychological, we must embrace the more penetrating models of community engagement in end of life care.

Professionally led inpatient units encounter serious demographic, geographical, technical and financial barriers when built in resource poor settings. They are inadequate to provide the care required for the large numbers who need it, meaning services are accessible only by the few. The only solution to achieve meaningful care for the great majority of those with chronic and incurable illnesses is to provide it in their communities, on their doorsteps, where even the poor and debilitated can access it. This model translates to affluent settings, where inpatient units are often inadequate to provide care that truly enhances the quality of life of the dying person and their family. The dying person cannot be viewed in isolation from their family, friends and community. Whilst symptom control by doctors is essential, medical professionals can never address the myriad of social and existential problems that those facing death must contend with.

To address these concerns, communities must be engaged and empowered to help find solutions to the problems they face. This book explores projects throughout the world that have endeavoured to do just that. Chapter 1 sets the historical context for the alliance of public health and palliative care, and Chapter 2 explores in more detail the conceptual congruence between the two fields. Chapter 3 develops the concept of 'illness trajectories' to understand people's dynamic and evolving experiences at the end of life. Chapters 4, 5, and

6 provide overviews of a public health approach on a country or continent-wide level. Different examples from Australia, the UK and Africa illustrate the diverse and innovative ways in which a public health approach can subtly and overtly influence the development of the palliative care agenda. The subsequent chapters provide practice examples from a diverse range of settings. Chapter 7 provides an account of the prolific spread of palliative care through the southern Indian state of Kerala, due in large part to the embracing by local communities of concepts of locally delivered and comprehensive care for the needy. Chapter 8 looks at how the community can be engaged in the contrasting inner city setting of east London, whilst Chapter 9 describes an initiative in Japan, where local schools, businesses and health and social care organizations are working together to create 'dementia friendly communities' where those with dementia can live safely in the community whilst continuing to contribute to the society in which they live. Chapter 10 looks at the transferability of a model from an urban developed world context to a rural developing world setting. Chapter 11 assesses a longstanding initiative, run in partnership with St Christopher's Hospice in London, linking children from local schools with patients from the hospice. There, using creative arts, myths around death, dying and the hospice can be challenged. Finally, Chapter 12 looks at a nascent palliative care service in the South American country of Ecuador, where it was recognized from the outset that care must go beyond simply the provision of services. The public health agenda has evolved alongside palliative care provision, leading to important developments in policy and legislation, in parallel with community development and medical support.

This book is intended as a handbook and practical guide for those wishing to initiate models of palliative care which engage local communities to improve the provision of palliative care for patients and their families. The appendices include resources and guidance about how to initiate services in a range of settings and stages of development. They include information on how to begin engaging with local community groups or to start a service, and an example of a national policy for a public health approach to palliative care.

By illustrating the many and diverse models of community engagement in palliative care that exist around the world, this book hopes to inspire its readers and to support new and innovative initiatives in the care of the dying and their families, friends and communities.

LS, SK and AK
London, 2011

Acknowledgements

We would like to thank the numerous organizations that have allowed us to reproduce their material for the appendices: the Government of Kerala, the Neighbourhood Network in Palliative Care, the 100 Member Committee, La Trobe University Palliative Care Team and Palliative Care Australia. Appendix 2 is reproduced with permission of the publisher (www.informaworld.com) from 'Charter for the Normalisation of Dying, Death and Loss' by E. Clark, J. Dawes, L.A. DeSpelder, Allan Kellehear *et al.*, *Mortality*, Vol. 10:2, pp. 157–161 (2005). We would also like to extend our thanks to the participants of the First International Conference on Public Health and Palliative Care, held in Calicut, Kerala in January 2009.

1 Public health and palliative care

An historical overview

Allan Kellehear and Libby Sallnow

What is public health?

The twentieth century has seen dramatic improvements in mortality rates and life expectancy; an achievement widely attributed to 'public health advances' rather than to clinical medicine. But the ubiquitous use of the term 'public health' can cause confusion, as much public health practised today bears little resemblance to that practised by the founders of this movement in the mid-nineteenth century. Public health is concerned with the health of people on a population level. It aims to reduce mortality and morbidity and improve the health of communities, cities or nations. As public health focuses on major killers or disease burdens, it must evolve as they change.

Health is influenced by more than just biomedical factors and thus public health is linked to the prevalent social, political and economic influences on health. Public health is usually defined in terms of its aims: to reduce disease and improve health. As public health does not adhere to a particular theoretical framework or specific methodology, tensions can exist between different areas. It is currently said to be facing a crossroads (Beaglehole and Bonita 2004) but, in order to understand the current tensions, it is important to acknowledge the history of the movement, as the struggles and successes of the past inform many of the current conflicts.

The history of public health

The importance of maintaining the health of a population has been recognized by governments and doctors alike since the time of Hippocrates. Although some changes implemented by the Romans and Greeks would now be classed as public health measures, the concerted study of public health as a discipline can be traced to the time of the Industrial Revolution. Rapid urbanization and the development of industry on a large scale presented sudden threats to health and new disease burdens. In addition to this, the traditional means of coping with illness, injury and dying were stripped away as people left their rural communities where strong support networks for the needy and vulnerable had been built up.

Governments began to focus specifically on threats to health, primarily as they were seen to have an influence on economic productivity and social order. The first public health studies were broad demographic studies of mortality rates in different districts and from these an appreciation of the social and environmental determinants of disease grew. In France, in 1821, a surgeon, Rene Louis Villermé, examined the health implications of a large study of mortality rates carried out in Paris.

Searching for a factor that correlated with the high rates seen in certain districts, he found that the strongest by far was income (Porter 1999). In the UK, at approximately the same time, people were becoming increasingly dissatisfied with the Poor Laws, a set of measures devised to support those who could not work. It was felt they were an unnecessary expenditure and in 1834 a report was commissioned into the causes of poverty and the need for the Poor Laws. This enquiry was chaired by Edwin Chadwick, a committed follower of the emerging school of thought of Utilitarianism. The link was made between poverty and ill health but it was believed that disease caused poverty, rather than poverty influencing disease (Hamlin 1994). It was felt that if you removed causes of disease, resolution of poverty would follow. In accordance with the established theories of disease, such as the theory of miasma, the idea that diseases are spread by the gases emitted from rotting matter, the recommendations were narrow in scope and reflected the prevalent reductionist approach to health. New sewer systems and waste disposal schemes were installed but no attempts were made to address the other causes of poverty. The revolution heralded by the germ theory later in the nineteenth century served only to compound this reductionist approach and the remit of public health was narrowed further.

In 1847, a typhoid epidemic broke out in the Prussian province of Silesia. The government was concerned as it was impacting on the profits from the mining industry and Rudolf Virchow, a young doctor, was sent to investigate the causes. He had been influenced by the work of Chadwick and Villermé and produced a report detailing the social causes for the outbreak and recommending better pay and working hours, housing and diet and a joint committee of lay people and professionals to monitor and organize the relief efforts (Waitzkin 2006). He was dismissed after his report was filed but the experience shaped Virchow's view of disease and he maintained that every disease has two causes: the pathological and the political.

Public health in the eighteenth and nineteenth century is often referred to as the 'Golden Age' of public health, when rapid improvements in mortality rates were made and control over many diseases was achieved. Sanitary reform and legislative action were the basis for public health measures in the mid- to late eighteenth century, with dramatic improvements in mortality rates seen in many areas (Szreter 1988). The germ theory heralded a new era, which overshadowed the older, environmental approaches. A focus on transmission, isolation and targeted antimicrobial therapies caused public health to become colonized with medical professionals and the social reformers were gradually squeezed out. Public health slowly became a specialty allied to medicine. The twentieth century posed a dramatically different set of challenges to public health. The previous century had been dominated by conditions such as cholera, tuberculosis and malaria exacting a high death toll. The epidemiological transition to non-communicable diseases in the twentieth century in the developed world meant public health needed to find new methods to approach the health problems presented by these diseases. Aetiologies were not easily elucidated and were multifactorial. A single biological factor was not responsible, meaning prevention strategies had to look outside the contemporary scientific sphere.

The new public health

The broadening of the 'host-agent' paradigm that had long dominated public health prompted those in public health to again re-examine the causes of disease. In the UK, a report was commissioned in the 1970s to look at inequalities in health. The Black report, written by Sir Douglas Black, found that a gradient favouring the higher socioeconomic classes existed in most health indicators. This disparity persisted despite the National Health Service providing medical care free at the point of delivery (Davey Smith *et al.* 2001). This and other similar realizations around the world meant that the social determinants of disease were once again considered when looking at causes and prevention of disease.

In Canada, this appreciation of the wider social determinants of disease was formalized in 1974 with the 'Health Field Concept'. The then health minister, Marc Lalonde, argued that four elements were involved in determining health outcomes: human biology, environment, lifestyle and health services (Lalonde 1974). This prompted an examination of lifestyle and environmental factors that individuals could control that would then influence health. Although useful in broadening the scope of public health, this was later criticized as creating a culture of 'blaming the victim', as many of these factors were in fact beyond an individual's control.

The Alma-Ata Declaration of 1978 by the World Health Organization (WHO) took this a step further. In order for comprehensive primary care services to be successful in improving the health of communities, the services needed to be appropriate and sustainable. The key part of this was participation of the local community. Services should be developed in partnership with local people, meaning they would be able to accurately address the needs of the people they were serving. This suggestion of health interventions being done *with* people rather than *on* people is one of the central themes of the new public health. The Alma-Ata Declaration was followed in 1986 by the Ottawa Charter for Health Promotion (see Box 1.1). This was again put forward by the WHO and it proposed a new model for addressing health, defining it in a positive way, rather than simply the absence of disease. In addition to individual lifestyle factors involved in determining health, there were other, more structural or ecological factors that also need to be tackled in order to see any real health gains. For example, health education and empowerment needs to be followed by legislative action such as seatbelt laws or a ban on cigarette advertising.

Box 1.1 The Ottawa Charter

1   Building healthy public policy
2   Creating supportive environments
3   Strengthening community action
4   Developing personal skills
5   Re-orientating health services

Source: adapted from WHO (1986)

The new discipline of health promotion was built on the participatory notion of health, namely that the very people whose health was affected often had the answers about how to solve the problems. The professional dominance of those from outside assuming they knew best for a community was challenged and this set the new public health apart from previous initiatives.

Hospices, poor houses and the development of palliative care

The adoption of the term 'hospice' by the early workers in palliative care in the 1960s both acknowledged the history of institutions caring for pilgrims, travellers and the poor when sick, but also reflected a new philosophy. The significant historical, cultural and religious overtones contained in the word 'hospice' mean it is not a neutral term and it has been used to describe widely different, if not contradictory, institutions over time. The history of hospices through time reflects the parallel developments in scientific, religious and political arenas.

In the early uses of the term, in the Middle Ages, 'hospice' was synonymous with 'hospital', as places for the sick to reside. The lack of any formal medical presence meant the distinction between investigation and treatment or supportive care was not made. In the affluent classes, medical care was provided in the home and thus the majority of the patients in the early hospices were the poor and homeless. With the advent of the Crusades and religious pilgrimages, large numbers of people were displaced from home. They required shelter and support when they became unwell whilst travelling, and these were met by the early religious hospices. Often run by monks or nuns, they were based on the Christian ethic of care for the needy and there was an emphasis on meeting spiritual needs (Saunders and Ross 2001). With the Reformation, many of these religious hospices were disbanded and, as the profession of medicine began to develop, a distinction between hospices and hospitals developed. Many hospitals instated a policy of not admitting incurable or dying patients, emphasizing that they were places of cure (von Gunten 2005).

The Industrial Revolution caused great social upheaval. The large number of people living in the newly created cities had left behind their communities and traditional means of support. When they became ill or homeless they needed to look for new, alternative means of support. The workhouses provided the employment for the majority of the new inhabitants of the cities. Living in slums and working in dangerous conditions, the mortality and morbidity rates were high and traditional family roles changed as all were required to work in the factories.

New provision was required to house the poor who could no longer work or who were dying. The workhouse infirmaries or poor houses were the solution to this problem. Created simply to house this section of society, there was little medical provision and no ethos of care of the individual. In Spain in the eighteenth century, the Royal Hospice in Madrid was said to act as both an alms house and a jail. Legislative change aimed to contain poverty, and undesirable elements of society were sent to the hospice and kept there under armed guard. These associations have been maintained, with the current meaning of a hospice in-patient, *hospiciano*, still denoting extreme poverty (Nunez Olarte 1999). Thus the old understanding of the term 'hospice' centred around ideas of containment (Humphreys 2003) – containment of disease, undesirable aspects of society and pollution, as this was seen as synonymous with disease. This institutionalized view of end of life care – to view death and dying as polluting experiences to be 'contained' – reflected the prevalent ideas in public health at the time.

The theories of contagion and miasma suggested that pollution and poverty should be kept away from the healthy, to protect them, and there was no consideration of more inclusive strategies to address the root causes and integrate the different aspects of society. The development of the modern hospice movement has its roots in this tradition – a commonly unacknowledged insight into the sociology of health policies for end of life care. Institutions were built to house the dying, to set them apart from the community (Abel 1986). Although they were intended to serve the terminally ill of the community, they were not involved with it and this could also be seen as an effort to 'contain' the dying from the wider society. The paradigm is now gradually being shifted to take a broader view of the dying and terminally ill.

Influenced by the ideas of new public health and community empowerment, the boundaries between institutions and communities are being broken down and a more participatory, interactive collaboration is being developed: moving away from the focus on disease to a more positive understanding of health; away from containment of pollution and poverty to emphasizing social and collective responsibility. A public health approach to palliative care today includes all these elements and is part of the broader and global health promotion movement.

The emergence of community development in health promotion

As mentioned earlier, in 1986 the WHO released the Ottawa Charter for Health Promotion. This charter became a watershed of ideas for the 'new' public health. Though new ideas of public health had already made the association between the idea of physical settings and environments to social settings and environments, the mode of working in these quite different ecologies was largely unknown or unprecedented. There were many public health workers who merely felt that social environments – individuals and groups going about their everyday business of work, play or worship – should be 'targeted' and changed with 'interventions'. The problem of cancer, for example, like the problem of polluted drinking water or poor sanitation, should simply be subject to the same interests in surveillance, education and then appropriate health services.

The Ottawa Charter was among the first modern public health documents that challenged this didactic, professional dominance model. Its five principles advocated the building of public policies that supported health (as opposed to only disease intervention) but it was clear that this meant the need to 'create supportive environments', to 'strengthen community action', as well as to develop personal skills and re-orient health services. In meeting these new and somewhat radically different goals, the new public health was to be 'participatory'. This was no set of public health initiatives that added to the list of things that we, as professionals, *do TO others*. The new approach to public health was that health and social care was a collection of changes to enhance health and safety that we *do WITH others*.

In this subtle change of policy language, a new and rather novel set of assumptions had crept in. It had long been assumed in the 'old' public health model that professional health workers knew best. People who were not 'trained' in health knowledge characteristic of academic subjects such as medicine, nursing or public health were 'lay' people. Lay people were largely ignorant of their own health because their knowledge about anatomy, biology, pathophysiology or clinical pharmacology were minimal or absent. The expertise, and therefore the authority and responsibility for surveillance and change, must emanate from professionals. It became rapidly apparent in the 1960s that there were severe limits and constraints on this approach and these assumptions.

Furthermore, public health research in diverse areas from occupational health and safety, sexual and mental health to cardiovascular and gastrointestinal medicine were uncovering the fact that many dimensions of an individual's health were not entirely under that individual's control. Moreover, individuals and groups had extensive experience concerning the barriers that needed to be overcome to access better health in their own work, family or sexual circles and environments. In other words, so-called 'lay' populations enjoyed their own 'expertise' because only they knew best HOW better health might be obtained because they were often more knowledgeable about what they were personally up against to achieve this. People often recognized the barriers to their own health goals, and were able to identify the supports needed to help them give up smoking, eat an improved diet or who to depend on in times of crisis or trauma. Recognition of this social fact meant that a partnership between health services and communities became essential to health promotion.

In matters to do with end of life care, the need to work with communities in designing their own ways to care for one another is an equally important aspect of a health promoting palliative care approach (Kellehear 1999, 2005). Within the personal and social experience of bereavement, those bereaved in the past often have substantial experience about what was helpful to them – or not. Within the experience of caring for an elderly relative with dementia or cancer, families and other personal carers often have a wealth of experience about what was helpful to them – or not. Among any community living with social difference – gay and lesbian members, migrants and refugees, those living with cancer or mental or physical disabilities to name only a few – lies a wealth of knowledge, experience and therefore 'expertise' about loss, grief, vulnerability and support.

A community development approach to end of life care both accepts and seeks to learn from such authoritative experience and people and to match and balance this with the more traditional but different kinds of expertise found among our health professionals. This subtle but all-important distinction still remains today as one of the more difficult and misunderstood areas of health promoting palliative care. The work of Rao and colleagues (2002, 2005; Gomez-Batiste 2005) illustrates this tension well. Rao and colleagues advocate a public health approach to end of life care but their emphasis is placed firmly on issues of 'raising awareness', public or patient education, communication needs, understanding cultural beliefs or 'access to support 'services'. The emphasis is clearly on attitude change and profession-led services and education. Less attention is paid to community change and community-led supports.

In a contrasting but complementary way, the work of Kumar (2007) places a health promotion approach squarely at the centre of his end of life care theory and practice. A participatory approach to end of life care in the Indian approach to palliative care in Kerala, for example, is to encourage communities to take both the lead and the key responsibilities for care in *partnership* with existing services (see Chapter 7).

On the other hand, Australian contexts of affluence, gentrification and urban work cultures do not easily lend themselves to such major responsibilities. The long-standing cultural expectation is to rely on services, greater quality supports, and supports that work seamlessly as part of a broader public health approach to end of life care. Such approaches to support are made possible by health promoting, participatory and community development approaches (Kellehear and Young 2007; Kellehear and O'Connor 2008). Hence the community development approach to end of life care grows directly from the health promotion imperative to create participatory relations, to encourage not simply 'attitude' but real social changes to the quality of services and supports that dying people and their families encounter. The health promotion emphases are not confined to attitudes but also actions; not only patient learning from professionals but professional learning from communities; not only 'what we can do' but also 'what we can do together'. Health promotion initiatives can and do work in national contexts such as Australia. Chapter 4 provides an overview of how some of these ideas have taken root in these cultural and service contexts.

The social importance of community development in end of life care

There are two reasons why a community development approach is socially important to the way we care for dying people, those who care for them and those who are left bereaved after their loved ones die. These reasons are to increase and enhance quality of life for both dying people and their carers, and to increase access to both end of life care support and services. Such reasons apply whether we are addressing end of life care practice issues in affluent contexts such as the US, Britain or Australia (where increasing quality of life is a stated priority), or resource-poor areas of the world such as Africa, India or Central Asia, where access to basic support and services is the priority.

In the first case of increasing quality of life in affluent societies, governments in these kinds of countries now face more than ever before a declining budget capacity to fund significant service expansion. The need for a so-called 'whole person' approach to care – one that demands that health authorities take spiritual and social matters seriously for dying people – can only mean two things. Either we employ more professionals or services in social work, pastoral care, chaplaincy or counselling; or we look to a broader public health approach that seeks to strengthen community ability to provide these kinds of supports. A third approach – the use of hospice volunteers – has been limited and of limited value. Volunteers in the UK and Australia, for example, have frequently been employed to offer menial services such as reading or transport, under the authority and surveillance of professionals and their hospices. Alternatively, volunteers have been used to fundraise or help spread information about local hospice and palliative care services. Their 'expertise' as members of the community has played a lesser role. Since funding more professionals to provide support outside of any institutional area such as a hospice must only have a limited future and even more limited capacity, the only alternative seems to be to strengthen community capacity for this kind of support.

Although there are several community development models – from hiring community development workers to forming partnership with community-based organizations to directly working with schools, workplaces or media sources – the challenge to date is achieving a critical mass of awareness that this is the actual challenge before us. The policy emphasis continues to linger about possible 'service' offerings that might still be feasible if more funding or redeployment were possible. Yet, sometimes only a few metres or miles away exist public health or community health services that have been building community capacity for HIV prevention and care, women's and children's health, or have been developing community-based initiatives for changing workplace and recreational practices that strengthen community resources for the disabled. Such long and established experience begs a new relationship with end of life care.

On the other hand, for these public health colleagues and services death and loss are sometimes publicly held up for all to see as threatening and frightening experiences to avoid. Death and dying are used in this way as symbolic prompts to move behaviour towards health promotion and active help-seeking. In other words, death and dying have frequently been employed by traditional public health colleagues and campaigns to frighten people into health promotion practices. But dying is living, and is not to be conflated with death. Those people living with dying have health promotion needs that speak to their potential to live fuller and satisfying lives even in the shadow of death.

Beyond the limited storylines of past public health messages about life, health and death, public health workers frequently do not see that living with dying, caring for dying and living with loss do, in fact, have significant morbidities and mortalities that are preventable or amenable to harm reduction strategies. Dying is also a complex set of journeys – it is not one type of physical or social trajectory but several. Chapter 3 demonstrates the need to understand these complexities so that we do not oversimplify the needs of the dying and our health promotion approach to them. Community development approaches to support the different needs of different kinds of dying have significant possibilities for goals as diverse as suicide prevention, the prevention of discrimination or social isolation, and or the enhancement of knowledge and practices that help people share social burden and personal loss (see Chapter 10 for an Australian health promotion approach to helping the carer which can help the dying person).

In resource-poor countries, it is often not feasible or practical to continue to build hospices. In policy terms alone, it is not clear that fundraising for often-expensive in-patient facilities should take priority over cheaper, more penetrating community initiatives. Constructing more buildings is a narrow view of increasing access (see Chapter 5, which addresses the African palliative care challenges). It is NOT the case that in-patient services are less important than community initiatives but that in-patient services might more practically become an outgrowth of community-based supports and services rather than the reverse (see Chapters 8, 11 and 12 for services that are able or are aiming to employ health promotion approaches as essential adjuncts to their traditional in-patient approaches to care in the UK and Ecuador).

Aside from matters of financial cost, the practical reality of a hospice or in-patient palliative care services in an existing hospital is that usually the majority of the rural population cannot travel there. In Eastern Europe and Central Asia, for example, the cost of a motor vehicle or its running costs make travel to a major city impossible or impractical for most. The other problem with immobile in-patient facilities is that dying and its care must necessarily be endured away from home or the homelands, again, specifically for the majority who live in rural areas. Such physical dislocation encourages social dislocation as other friends and family are not able to travel or stay for significant lengths of time with the dying person and their direct carers. In all these instances of service-driven initiatives or of prioritizing in-patient services, both the epidemiological adequacy and geographical coverage of this end of life care strategy are inadequate. Only a broader public health approach that places community development at its policy and practice heart can meet the twin challenges of distance and whole person care. This is another reason why 'public health initiatives' also go by the alternative label of 'population health' approaches.

For resource-poor countries the challenge for well-meaning foreigners with affluent service-culture mentalities, and for locals who equate buildings and professionals with images of modern, superior care, this is a difficult message to sell. However, to be fair, in international and historical terms, a public health approach to end of life care has been and remains a difficult message to sell anywhere. The culturally powerful – but valid – image of the hospital and the health professional as effective responses to acute crises of health has spilled uncontrollably into the management of chronic illness, ageing and dying. Remarkably if unbelievably, this is so despite the fact that these heroic early images sit paradoxically with other latter images of decrepitude and neglect in nursing institutions, technological over-servicing and brinkmanship in hospital-based end of life care, and increasing levels of social isolation amid economic plenty. Chapter 9 describes alternatives taken by the Japanese to shown that such predicaments and outcomes are not inevitable, even in affluent contexts. Yet, the sociological background we have discussed here remains fertile ground for several other barriers to the uptake of a public health, community-based approach.

Challenges for the future

There are three great challenges that face the current rising interest in public health approaches to end of life care and they are all inter-related. For those of us who are interested in a health promoting palliative care or a health promoting aged care, the main challenge appears to be the inability, the reluctance or the refusal to understand key health promotion concepts and apply these as they were originally designed. As Rosenberg argues in Chapter 2, there is a common and all too widespread tendency to interpret health promotion as mere health education. Equally, many palliative care services continue to see community development as simply community work – things that services do *to* communities rather than things services do *with* communities. Power-sharing is awkward and the ability to articulate, let alone recognize, community authority in matters to do with end of life care comes slowly. There remains a strong desire to interpret health promotion as yet another 'service' performed by professionals on 'patients and their families'. An understanding that public health approaches, in the health promotion sense, does not have 'patients' is poorly understood and – for many professionals – disempowering. This problem underscores the second challenge facing those of us with public health interests.

Though there is rising interest in the public health approach to end of life care, training for this re-orientation is poor or absent. Though strong experiments and practice examples exist in Australia and India these are not easily accessed by practitioners in the UK, the US or Hong Kong, for example. The desire to learn about health promoting palliative care is not matched by training programmes, additional funding or inter-sectoral co-operation between end of life care services and mainstream public health services. Public health workers still view death and dying as failure and see little or no role for themselves in end of life care. Palliative care workers continue to see themselves in an old public health tradition and do not seek to align themselves with the ideas of the new public health. Of those who do wish to align themselves, many have neither the training nor the political imagination to forge new connections with their public health colleagues. As Steve Conway observes in Chapter 6 about the new UK End of Life Care Strategy, the phrase 'public health' appears weakly in the form of another allied idea, that of 'public awareness'. This situation will continue unless one further challenge is addressed.

The public health sector – those responsible for our community campaigns for tobacco and alcohol control, cycling and workplace safety programmes, our obesity and sexual health programmes to name just a few – need to enter the end of life care arena. Those of us in palliative care, aged care, bereavement care, emergency and disaster management, or intensive care, need to learn and be supported by those in health care who understand and have practice experience with community development, health promotion, critical reflection, legislative change, policy reform, and social and political change. Without their support, active encouragement and partnership end of life care will remain in its institutionalized origins and fail to understand, less embrace, the social reality of dying, death and loss as a community experience. And that would be a major and ongoing loss for us all.

References

Abel, E.K. (1986) The hospice movement: Institutionalising innovation, *International Journal of Health Services*, 16(1): 71–85.

Beaglehole, R. and Bonita, R. (2004) *Public Health at the Crossroads*, Cambridge: Cambridge University Press.

Davey Smith, G., Dorling, D. and Shaw, M. (eds) (2001) *Poverty, Inequality and health in Britain, 1800–2000: A Reader*, Bristol: Policy Press.

Gomez-Batiste, X. (2005) Catalonia WHO Palliative Care Demonstration Project at 15 years, *Journal of Pain and Symptom Management*, 33(5): 584–90.

Hamlin, C. (1994) *State medicine in Great Britain*, in Porter, D. (ed.) *The History of Public Health and the Modern State*, Amsterdam: Rodopi.

Humphreys, C. (2003) Tuberculosis, poverty and the first 'hospices' in Ireland, *European Journal of Palliative Care*, 10(4): 164–7.

Kellehear, A. (1999) *Health Promoting Palliative Care*, Melbourne: Oxford University Press.

Kellehear, A. (2005) *Compassionate Cities: Public health and end of life care*, London: Routledge.

Kellehear, A. and O'Connor, D. (2008) Health promoting palliative care: A practice example, *Critical Public Health*, 18(1): 111–15.

Kellehear, A. and Young, B. (2007) Resilient Communities, in Monroe, B. and Oliviere, D. (eds) *Resilience in palliative care: Achievements in adversity*, Oxford: Oxford University Press.

Kumar, S. (2007) Kerala, India: A Regional Community-Based Palliative Care Model, *Journal of Pain and Symptom Management*, 33(5): 623–7.

Lalonde, M. (1974) A New Perspective on the Health of Canadians, Ottawa: National Health and Welfare.

Nunez Olarte, J.M. (1999) Care of the dying in 18th century Spain – the non-hospice tradition, European Journal of Palliative Care, 6(1): 23–6.

Porter, R. (1999) The greatest benefit to mankind; A medical history of humanity from antiquity to the present, London: Fontana Press.

Rao, J.K., Alongi, J., Anderson, L.A., Jenkins, L., Stokes, G.A. and Kane, M. (2005) Development of public health priorities for end-of-life initiatives, American Journal of Preventative Medicine, 29(5): 453–60.

Rao, J.K., Anderson, L.A. and Smith, S.M. (2002) End of life is a public health issue, American Journal of Preventative Medicine, 23(3): 215–20.

Saunders, Y. and Ross, J. (2001) St Joseph's Hospice: then and now, European Journal of Palliative Care, 8(3): 115–18.

Szreter, S. (1988) The importance of social intervention in Britain's mortality decline. 1850–1914: a re-interpretation of the role of public health, Social Science and Medicine, 1(1): 1–37.

von Gunten, C. (2005) The Academic Hospice, Annals of Internal Medicine, 143(9): 655–58.

Waitzkin, H. (2006) One and a Half Centuries of Forgetting and Rediscovering: Virchow's Lasting Contributions to Social Medicine, Social Medicine, 1(1): 5–10.

World Health Organization (1986) Ottawa Charter for Health Promotion.

World Health Organization and UNICEF (1978) Primary Health Care: Report of the International Conference on Primary Health Care. Alma-Ata USSR. 6–12 September, 1978. Geneva: WHO.

2 'But we're already doing it!'

Examining conceptual blurring between health promotion and palliative care

John Rosenberg

Introduction

Over the past decade, an increasing number of palliative care service providers have attempted to integrate health promotion into their organisational practice. A key factor in the success of this endeavour has been the recognition by these providers of the conceptual 'fit' between two seemingly disparate approaches to health care. When informed of the elements of health promotion, palliative care professionals have expressed their recognition in their declaration: 'But we're already doing it!' (Rosenberg 2007).

Yet it appears that this association between the two suggests that health promotion in palliative care organisations is being understood in poorly defined ways. 'Health promotion' can be incorrectly assumed to be synonymous with 'health education'; 'death education' can be understood to be synonymous with providing information about palliative care resources. Whilst these activities may be worthwhile within themselves, their presence in the activities of an organisation does not constitute the practice of health promoting palliative care (HPPC) (Kellehear 1999).

The relatively recent return of palliative care services into mainstream health care systems has included systemic, public health approaches to the governance of the care and support of people at the end of life (Palliative Care Australia 2005; Scott 1992). These approaches represent a departure from the early origins of the modern hospice movement, where freestanding, independent hospices with home-based outreach were a common service configuration; typically these services were voluntarily sequestered from mainstream health care until more recently (Howarth 2007). However, there are misconceptions about these public health approaches and a blurring of the key concepts in integrating a HPPC approach.

Key concepts in health promotion and palliative care

Palliative care and health promotion have a great deal in common (Rosenberg and Yates 2010). Both emerged in the latter half of the twentieth century from dissatisfaction with the dominant biomedical approach to health care, which was criticised for its reductionist and mechanistic understanding of human disease and illness (Baum 2008) and for the removal of the sick person from their social, cultural and spiritual contexts within which they experience illness (Bunton and MacDonald 2002). Yet tacitly we can acknowledge that health, and death, are both experienced by people as deeply embedded in their lived experience.

Palliative care

Contemporary palliative care is derived from a 'small rebellion' (Connor 1998, p. xiii), which sought to restore 'an holistic approach to patient care, the family as the focus of care, and importance of multidisciplinary collaboration on a day to day basis' (Hockley 1997 p. 84). Palliative care is underpinned by numerous key concepts, which include its aim to:

- Affirm life and regards dying as normal.
- Integrate the psychological and spiritual aspects of care.
- Offer comprehensive support to promote quality of life.
- Offer support systems to help patients live as actively as possible until death.

(World Health Organization 2008)

These key concepts *for practice* clearly situate the dying person squarely in their lived reality. Dying is not simply a medical event, but a profoundly personal, interpersonal and communal one. The planning and provision of support by the health care professions, therefore, must be responsive to this view. It is clear to see, then, that the support of dying people and their families is the responsibility of both the health care professions and the communities in which the dying person lives:

> The experiences of serious illness, dying, care giving, grieving and death cannot be completely understood within a medical framework alone. These events are personal, but also fundamentally communal. Medical care and health services constitute essential components of a community's response, but not its entirety.
>
> (Byock *et al.* 2003, p. 760)

This understanding of palliative care as a holistic and contextualised endeavour underscores that death is viewed as a part of life, understands the notion of the whole person experiencing terminal illness, and views the patient's family as 'client'.

By creating environments of care where these core values could be practised, these concepts became accepted over time as the preferred method of caring for dying people. There were early indications that specialised hospice programs were more effective in relieving the suffering caused by pain and other symptoms

(Mor *et al.* 1998). The recognition of *palliative medicine* as a specialty in the UK in 1987 (Lewis 2007) was an acknowledgment of the particular set of medical skills required to treat the dying person. The approach to care of the dying that was offered by specialist interdisciplinary palliative care teams was increasingly viewed as the optimal approach to end of life care, where places of specialised care were provided for a few, and clinical consultation for the many was provided to an even smaller number. The 'small rebellion' had evolved into a substantial parallel path to mainstream health care.

The difficulty that arose from this was that this 'boutique' approach to care of the dying provided support to only a small minority of its potential patients; in one location in Australia, specialised palliative care was noted to be primarily provided to relatively younger people with cancer, and by no means all of them (Hunt and Maddocks 1997) and similar criticisms have been made in the UK (Douglas 1992). In practice, people dying with non-malignant disease or the very old were largely excluded from access to specialised palliative care services. In some parts of the US, it has been suggested that the palliative care movement substantially – although not universally – failed in responding to the need for the care of people dying from AIDS as it emerged as a new life-limiting disease (Beresford 1993). There were concerns that this specialisation may also place the original core values of palliative care at risk, with its practitioners becoming little more than 'symptomatologists' (Kearney 1992) as they responded to requests for intervention in difficult cases. The need for a broader scope of practice was increasingly evident.

Fortunately, a growing awareness of the potential for a complementary coexistence between mainstream health care and palliative care arose:

> While the early hospices had often sought to stand outside the constraints of health care planners and their associated bureaucracies, the maturation of the movement was to bring about a growing interdependence with the wider structures of health care delivery.
>
> (Clark *et al.* 1997, p. 60)

This reintegration into mainstream health care acknowledged that the care of the dying person was an important part of *all* health professionals' practice and that palliative care should be regarded as *an integral part of health care* for many patients (UK Department of Health 1995). As such, it was not simply the responsibility of individual practitioners or sole hospices, but of the health care systems of countries or their jurisdictions. The World Health Organization's (WHO) *Cancer Relief and Palliative Care Report* (1990) emphasised the need for a systematic, planned approach to the provision of care for people dying from cancer and this represents an early and significant attempt to influence the utilisation of public health approaches in palliative care delivery.

This mainstreaming has brought both benefits and risks to the key concepts of palliative care. By conforming to the regulatory norms of health care systems, palliative care is at risk of fulfilling Kearney's (1992) fear that the spiritual and social realms will be lost; care of the dying could be reduced to little more than a set of medico-nursing interventions provided at the expense of psychological and social interventions (Kellehear 1999).

Health promotion

Like palliative care, health promotion emerged in response to a perceived over-emphasis on disease and its diagnosis, treatment and cure. Again, it seemed that the dominant biomedical approach to health care failed to adequately embrace whole population issues and the complex interrelationships between the physical, psychological and social components of health and wellbeing (Bunton and MacDonald 2002). Unlike palliative care, the proponents of health promotion formed a more structured, global movement whose key concepts were integrated more quickly into health care systems.

The Ottawa Charter for Health Promotion originally defined health promotion as 'the process of enabling people to increase control over, and to improve, their health' (WHO 1986, p. 1). It described the highly contextualised nature of health and wellbeing, where the determinants of health are based upon a broad range of physical, social and environmental factors. Notably, the Ottawa Charter overtly declared that responsibility for the promotion of health rests not simply with the health sector but with governments, social and economic sectors, industry and media, and communities themselves. The Ottawa Charter famously provided a framework to achieve these goals in its five key action areas (see Box 1.1). The implementation of multiple, concurrent strategies in each of these key action areas is based upon the premise that people, and the communities in which they live, are central players in obtaining satisfactory states of health and not merely the passive recipients of health services; enabling people to achieve their full potential for health requires their engagement in the strategies being implemented (Baum 2008). In so doing, people will bring with them the social, cultural, spiritual and social elements of their experiences of health and illness. Subsequent WHO Health Promotion statements have reiterated and built upon the Ottawa Charter's original key concepts; *The Jakarta Declaration on Leading Health Promotion into the 21st Century* (World Health Organization 1997) re-emphasised the need for strategies beyond the health sector to optimise health and *The Bangkok Charter for Health Promotion in a Globalised World* (World Health Organization 2006) advocated placing the development of health at the centre of the global agenda, as a core responsibility of all governments and a key focus of communities.

It is clear that attempts to shape the attainment of health of individuals, families and communities were based on a broad range of health promotion strategies from local to global.

Health promoting palliative care

The seemingly paradoxical nature of suffering and the promotion of health may have been considered conceptually incompatible. Yet this only presents a paradigmatic difficulty when '...the perception of health [is] the absence of disease, and demands are made for medical services when treating ill health to have as their goal the absence of disease' (Pegg and Tan 2002, p. 25). The aim of health promotion to enable people to increase control over and to improve their health is not incompatible with the goals of palliative care to relieve pain and distress, and promote autonomy and self control, even in the absence of a likely cure (Pegg and Tan 2002).

Despite misgivings about conceptual compatibility, health promotion and palliative care have now been considered together for more than a decade. Evidence of this in the 1990s can be found (Faulkner 1993; Rosenberg 1992; Russell and Sander 1998; Scott 1992; Zeefe 1996); however, it was the seminal work of Australian sociologist Allan Kellehear (1999) that first provided a substantial and systematic examination of their compatibility. His contention was that '...if health is everyone's responsibility then it is also the responsibility of those living with a life-threatening or terminal illness as well as those who care for them' (Kellehear 1999, p. 31). This assertion reaffirms the statement within the Ottawa Charter in its key action area of developing personal skills that states the need for lifelong learning for people preparing themselves for *all of life's stages*.[1] Whilst dying as a life stage is not explicitly mentioned in the Ottawa Charter (or for many years thereafter in the health promotion literature), it is interesting to note this phrase in such a key document!

Whilst the centrality of holism as a response to the multidimensional nature of care at the end of life was present in the rhetoric of palliative care, Kellehear (1999) was critical of the overemphasis on the physical – and, to a lesser degree, psychological – symptomatology, whilst the social and spiritual domains remained ill-attended, as predicted by Kearney (1992). An HPPC approach, Kellehear asserted, addresses these underdeveloped aspects of conventional palliative care:

- Social and public health components
- The social aspects of care
- Early stage care
- Active treatment of disease
- Life-threatening illness (not just terminal care).

(Kellehear 1999)

Contemporary palliative care, Kellehear claimed, for the most part shows a 'palpable' (Kellehear 1999 p. 7) absence of social science and public health components leading to the neglect of the social domain within palliative care's own holistic framework. It falls short of providing truly 'social' care through its hybridisation of the psychological (i.e. individual) and social (i.e. collective) domains as 'psychosocial'. It fails to meet its own goal of providing support from the time of diagnosis and is primarily focussing its limited resources upon terminal care.

It is health promotion in the context of public health which Kellehear claimed addresses the risks – or actual inadequacies – in contemporary palliative care. He proposed five core concerns of HPPC:

- Provide education and information for health, death and dying.
- Provide social support at both personal and community levels.
- Encourage interpersonal reorientation.
- Encourage reorientation of palliative care services.
- Combat death-denying health policies and attitudes.

(Kellehear 1999)

Are there examples from real life that illustrate both philosophical and practical attempts to take a health promoting approach to palliative care? How do they demonstrate an ongoing attempt to clarify the conceptualisation of HPPC?

Conceptualising health promoting palliative care

Whilst the *practice* of public health and health promotion in palliative care has not always been systemically evident (Stjernsward 2007), the application of health promotion and public health approaches to palliative care have been *written about* by a number of scholars and practitioners. Attempts to integrate health promotion and palliative care demonstrate a growing awareness of the conceptual congruence between these two fields (Rosenberg and Yates 2010). Yet it is increasingly evident that this congruence has also brought at individual and organisational levels a lack of clarity, or conceptual blurring, of the key concepts underpinning HPPC.

Health education and information

Education has been viewed as the primary tool in informing and equipping members of the public for their inevitable involvement in death and dying (Gallagher 2001). This is seen as a strategy in reorientating health services by Zeefe (1996), who discussed the place of death education for staff, patients and families, and society more widely, as a pre-emptive strategy in equipping people with the life skills necessary for a healthy engagement with death and dying. This perspective reflects elements of health promotion in the Ottawa Charter in its use of empowerment and education to strengthen communities and develop personal skills of community members.

A Canadian author described an innovative public awareness and education tool that demonstrated the limited extent to which community engagement has been attempted. Gallagher's (2001) survey of trade-show visitors assessed respondents' knowledge of issues about dying and anticipated needs if they were to face a terminal illness. He identified varying levels of knowledge between health professionals and the general public about death, dying, care services, and euthanasia. A focus upon highly socially contextualised care included not simply the provision of clinical care, but information and education to 'overcome fear, relieve helplessness and promote health' (Scott 1992, p. 47).

Social support

The centrality of holism in the practice of a health promoting approach to palliative care was discussed by Buckley (2002), who viewed the process of adaptation experienced by dying people. Empowerment was a crucial attribute of the health promoting approach she proposed. In their study, Pegg and Tan (2002) similarly identified a link between suffering and quality of life, caused by lack of knowledge and limited empowerment. Weaver (2004) focused mostly on the needs of families during life-threatening illness and at the end of life, with its primary focus limited to promoting the health of the family unit. The dying patient was not seen as a recipient of health promotion strategies in this example.

The importance of support networks in the promotion of healthy bereavement was briefly described by Faulkner (1993) who integrated it into a risk-assessment tool titled 'Pre-Bereavement Predictors of Poor Outcome'. In particular, she considered the impact of absent or unsupportive family members, and detachment from traditional cultural and/or religious contexts on bereavement outcomes. Such use of preventative interventions in bereavement is commonplace today and is strongly congruent with the tenets of health promotion, given its potential to reorientate health services providing end of life care.

Skill development

Russell and Sander (1998) proposed a set of personal skills for professionals providing palliative care that demonstrated core elements of health promotion. *Enabling* requires both symptomatic expertise and social sensitivity to promote autonomy and control. *Advocacy* acknowledges the role of the health care professional to facilitate control back to the dying person. *Mediacy* influences the practices of the multidisciplinary team, and the wider context of health care. Russell and Sander also described the potential influence of nurses in reorientating health services in the care of dying people, in tandem with informing public policy. HPPC, they suggested, requires the development of a set of skills for professionals that could change the nature of health care practice.

Encourage interpersonal reorientation

In an attempt to reorientate occupational therapists' service provision to dying patients, vanderPloeg (2001) challenged her peers to extend their professional boundaries to optimise quality of life for their palliative care clients through the application of health promotion principles. She urged occupational therapists to optimise quality of life for palliative care clients through the use of a health pro-motion approach, and to provoke thought about individual practice rather than the wider issues of health care systems.

In a qualitative study of patients' perceptions of the therapeutic relationship with their nurses, another author proposed a 'definition of health promotion rel-evant to palliative nursing in the primary setting' (Richardson 2002, p. 432). Richardson described twelve patients' perceptions of the therapeutic relation-ship with their nurses, which enhanced their feelings of health and wellbeing. The therapeutic interventions contained in these relationships were modelled on health promotion principles, distinguishing between the therapeutic rela-tionship and the attention to the disease and its related symptoms.

Encourage reorientation of palliative care services

In an early attempt to articulate my nascent beliefs about how care of the dying could be done differently, I considered the inclusion of home-based palliative care services as integral to the Primary Health Care framework as described in the Declaration of Alma-Ata (World Health Organization 1978); I suggested that a 'healthy death for all' was a worthy goal for the provision of palliative care outside of institutional care (Rosenberg 1992).

Combat death-denying health policies and attitudes

In Canada, Scott (1992) used an epidemiological examination of life-threatening illnesses to show that a significant proportion of the population were not likely to survive their ailments, demonstrating an ongoing need for comprehensive and responsive palliative care. He was critical of an over-emphasis upon the prevention of cancer at the expense of education for the palliative care phase, in light of the prevalence of incurable cancer, and the suf-fering it caused. Scott proposed health promotion and public education as key strategies to address the escalating burden of suffering. He also claimed that this approach holds benefits for the cost effectiveness of palliative care, and sug-gested that the application of public health principles to end of life care could lead to an acceptance by government of the role of palliative care services in promoting public health.

More recently, Rao and colleagues (Rao *et al.* 2002, 2005) have provided one of the most substantive descriptions of public health and health promoting approaches to end of life care. They assert the need for the tangible inclusion of a public health approach in palliative care service planning. They argue that death awareness will be raised by emphasising the community's involvement in health, providing information and establishing partnerships; this empowerment of the community to contribute to debate of issues of quality of life at the end of life provides important foundations for end of life care. Rao *et al.* (2005) identi-fied nine clusters of public health activity that were directly relevant to the pro-vision of palliative care. Of these, five were identified as most feasible:

- Public education
- Patient, family and caregiver education
- Research, epidemiology and evaluation
- Professional education
- Policy and planning.

Importantly, each of these clusters was supplemented by a set of recommendations for action and demonstrated their application in the real world.

An Australian story

I conducted my doctoral research at an Australian palliative care service providing support to people choosing to die in their homes. As an organisation, the service had undertaken to integrate a HPPC approach as described in Kellehear's work. I studied the process of implementation of health promotion elements into the service's organisational structures and practices.

I asked staff and volunteers from the service about core concepts of health promotion, such as enabling, advocacy and mediacy (Russell and Sander 1998), and these were instantly recognisable to staff as core concerns for palliative care. There was an acceptance that health promotion and palliative care were, at least in principle, congruent: '*I think from the definitions I've read of health promoting palliative care, and the principles of it, and then hospice, they seem to fit together very closely . . .*' [director]. However for the most part, my examination of the transition being made to HPPC was framed by the five key action areas of the Ottawa Charter. Staff recognised some of these components in their palliative care organisation more readily than others. In particular, the two components that were most readily viewed as conceptually congruent were (a) *creating supportive environments* for consumers and for staff/volunteers, and (b) *developing personal skills*. Whilst other components of health promotion were less familiar to some respondents, they were, for the most part, viewed as appropriate inclusions in the work of palliative care. For example, strategies for *strengthening community action*, such as an annual street market, were seen as a fitting set of activities, but resource intensive.

With the health promotion component *building public policy*, there were some concerns expressed about the capacity of small, under-funded palliative care organisations like this service to participate, despite the relevance of this component. However, a greater impediment to the implementation this component of health promotion was an apparent lack of understanding of the scope of public policy. Whilst there were a few examples of participation in committees responsible in some part for policy development that impacts upon the provision of palliative care, an understanding of the scope of public policy was not strongly evident. This includes the notion of advocacy by palliative care service providers to governments for consumers' needs as an organisational responsibility rather than simply a characteristic of individual practitioners.

For the most part, however, they were able to grasp the conceptual congruence of all the elements after further consideration. This is well demonstrated in
this quotation from an interview with a staff member: '*It's going to be taken up
more readily and incorporated more readily because there's an alignment there … it's
not out of place with what is already in the philosophical thinking or with the work
practice …*' [staff member].

So there was a sense amongst the staff that, using the Ottawa Charter key
action areas, the service already demonstrated, to varying degrees, the components of health promotion in its practice. This dynamic state is illustrating in
Figure 2.1, which I have reproduced from my thesis.

However, this understanding led the staff to ask questions about the HPPC
approach. First, there were questions whether 'health promoting palliative care'
was just the latest jargon used to describe established and familiar elements of
palliative care practice, particularly the components of *creating supportive environments* and *developing personal skills*. Their familiarity with these elements
perhaps led to their perception that HPPC is a new term for established practices. This focus group participant asserted that '*… health promotion is what we
do. Someone has now come up and given it a name. I think all we can keep doing is
keep on at it.*' Whilst this claim showed conceptual congruence was strong, it
also demonstrates that participants in my research overlooked consideration of
the other key action areas of HPPC as equally important in end of life care and
integral to a HPPC model. As it was perceived as a new way of describing much
of what was already done, the integration of health promotion principles and
practice was viewed somewhat uncritically by some as already underway in the
service.

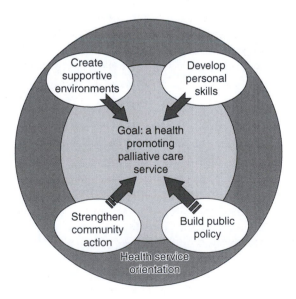

Figure 2.1 Integration of health promotion components

Second, questions were asked whether HPPC captured the 'core business' of the palliative care service – again, just a few respondents understood HPPC as a whole approach:

> ...while our core business remains home-based palliative care and education and support for families, it's also looking at affecting community attitudes to life and living, death and dying, funeral, the whole topic of death and preparing for death.
>
> (Director)

Others, however, viewed elements of HPPC as 'optional extras' for the conventional approach to palliative care service provision. The 'clinical' components were seen to be of a higher priority by these staff members than those focused upon community action. Significantly, those non-clinical services that can be 'delivered' as a 'service' – such as education – appeared more acceptable than those requiring robust engagement with the wider community.

These misgivings exceed Kellehear's (1999) prediction that HPPC might be viewed as simply 'an additional thing to do' (p. 23). This 'conceptual blurring' represents a risk to the effective implementation and practice of HPPC.

Achieving conceptual clarity

These examples demonstrate a paradoxical situation in the integration of HPPC in organisations. On the one hand, when the elements of health promotion are defined and explored by palliative care organisations, conceptual recognition seems to enable acceptance of HPPC as a valid approach to end of life care. On the other hand, however, the recognition of these elements has also led to both a sense of HPPC being an 'add-on' to clinical work, and a ready assumption of success in the integration of HPPC. This apparent ambivalence about elements of a HPPC model is worth considering in light of Kellehear's assertion that:

> Supplying health education or social support does not make a palliative care service health promoting any more than the provision of pain relief and a chaplain constitutes a conventional palliative care service. The practice of health promoting palliative care is a practice that embraces all the concerns together, in concert.
>
> (Kellehear 1999, p. 23)

This quote, the descriptions from the literature and my own study illustrate that conceptual blurring represents a great risk to the integration of HPPC. How then can conceptual blurring be avoided or remedied?

Let's return to the original components of the Ottawa Charter and pay specific attention to their translation into palliative care (Table 2.1). Taking 'Building public policies that support health' as an example, a number of authors have conceptually linked the practice of palliative care to public policy, arguing

Table 2.1 Translating the Ottawa Charter to palliative care

Key action areas to support health	Health promotion description	In palliative care organisations
Building public policies that support health	Health is on the agenda of all policy-makers, who must consider the health consequences of policy decisions. Obstacles to the adoption of healthy public policies need to be identified and removed.	Concerned with the participation of organisations in the development and/or uptake of public policy relating to palliative care and the support of dying people.
Creating supportive environments	Health cannot be separated from other societal goals. A sociological basis for health embraces the links between people and their environment.	Concerned with the ways in which organisations contribute to the creation of supportive environments to enhance wellbeing for consumers and employees of the palliative care service.
Strengthening community action	Communities set their own health priorities, make decisions, and plan and implement strategies to promote their empowerment. Community development enhances participation in, and direction of, health matters.	Related to the nature of the engagement of organisations with the wider community, beyond the recipients of palliative care services, to promote community action towards improved support of people at the end of life.
Developing personal skills	The enhancement of life skills through personal and social development promotes people exercising control over their health throughout life.	Concerned with organisations' participation in the development of personal skills to assist individuals to deal with issues around death and dying. Includes both health care professionals and primary caregivers.
Reorienting health services	Responsibility for health promotion within the health care system rests with all participants. Health services must move beyond clinical and curative services to support individuals and communities for a healthier life. Health research, professional education and training are necessary strategies for refocusing health services toward the needs of the whole person.	Related to the activities of organisations in reorienting their members to a health promoting approach, and has a particular focus on the holistic needs of its client population, and changes in organisational attitudes.

that death and dying are concerns for whole communities and society, and is consequently a concern of governments in their policy-making role. In turn, therefore, organisations that utilise a social model of health, such as that presented in HPPC, are validly able to include the development of public policy within their remit. This lends some support to the view that the end of life is indeed a public health concern, given the 'universal incidence' of death (Rao et al. 2002, p. 215). In Compassionate Cities, it is proposed a comprehensive policy framework for public health approaches to the end of life, including but not restricted to HPPC (Kellehear 2005). For example, Kellehear suggests the expression of compassion around issues of end of life translates into local health policies that recognise compassion as an ethical imperative, demonstrated in community education strategies including public forums, discussion groups, and crisis intervention. The responsibility of developing, implementing and evaluating these activities rests in partnerships between communities and organisations concerned with end of life issues. Notably, whilst this includes palliative care services, these public health strategies could be provided by grief and bereavement support services, aged care facilities, funeral directors, and other organisations concerned with end of life issues.

A genuine embracing of the social domain of dying through HPPC could lead to a paradigmatic shift in our many health systems and communities wherein dying people and their families are participants in the identification of need, and in the direction of care and support. These are clearly concepts close to both health promotion *and* conceptualisations of patient-centred care and holism so evident in the key concepts of palliative care. HPPC facilitates the preservation of social networks (including family) being seen as a priority for recipients of palliative care services and a validation of the desirability of social models of care (D'Onofrio and Ryndes 2003).

Create a critical mass for HPPC

Fundamental to the integration of health promotion with palliative care is the acceptability of the key concepts to the stakeholders in its implementation. Yet, in my study, the only respondents who demonstrated an understanding of the model as a whole were (a) the senior staff member charged with responsibility for the implementation of health promotion principles and practice in the service, and (b) a general staff member who had undertaken postgraduate studies in HPPC. That is to say, while other respondents demonstrated accurate understandings of specific components of health promotion, they did not demonstrate understanding of the HPPC model as both multifaceted and a whole approach. The suggestion of creating a critical mass of organisational personnel skilled and knowledgeable in health promotion (Whitelaw et al. 2006) may have addressed this.

Whole-of-organisation transition

To counter the risk of the compartmentalising of the elements of health promotion evident in my study and others' work, I believe a whole-of-organisation approach is optimal. There was some debate amongst respondents in my study as to whether a paradigmatic shift of this scale should – or even could – be implemented in a single, organisation-wide adjustment or rather, incrementally. In the service I studied the implementation of health promotion principles and practice was apparently piecemeal and, apart from a single planning document, seemed to lack a systematic, planned and organisation-wide perspective. This perhaps reflects limited understanding of the whole-of-organisation approach and the broader health promotion agenda. The fact that the site of my study struggled to formulate a comprehensive plan is indicative of the complex nature of the task and the multifaceted response it requires for success:

> ...we need a whole plan under the five strategies rather than doing one thing at a time. If you're changing public policy, you should be able to build sustainable communities at the same time ... you have to create awareness, so people are aware what palliative care is ... to effect public policy change, you have to get the voters to change public policy, so creating awareness is part of building sustainable communities.
>
> (Director)

Frameworks to facilitate such a plan have been suggested. For example, the HPPC practice guidelines developed by Kellehear and colleagues (Kellehear et al. 2003) provide a framework to guide palliative care organisations to undertake concrete health promoting activities, such as support groups, death education and policy development at governmental levels. One criterion of this framework is comprised of elements of a discrete community development program. The 'Big 7 Checklist' enables palliative care organisations to assess the alignment of end of life programs with public health and health promoting criteria (Salau 2006). This checklist includes prevention of social difficulties around death and loss through early intervention, participation of community members, the sustainability of program, and evaluation of their outcomes. An operational model for community based quality improvement in palliative care has been proposed by Byock et al. (2003) which demonstrated a method by which an organisation can establish the basis for its planned change, target priorities, develop and apply interventions and evaluate their effectiveness. It utilises the quality improvement cycle. With organisation-wide goals, it accommodates incremental implementation of strategies on an ongoing basis. In its emphasis upon a community approach to end of life care, it offers one approach to implementing HPPC.

Approaches other than whole-of-organisation have been suggested. Support for an incremental approach is found in work by Stajduhar et al. (2006), who chose a graduated approach in order to limit the risk of staff becoming overwhelmed by change of this magnitude. Others describe a lengthy, cyclical and complex process (Elwyn and Rhydderch 2002). Further evaluation of the effectiveness of these approaches is required.

Conclusion

This discussion has attempted to explore the phenomenon of conceptual blurring within HPPC, where the key concepts of both health promotion and palliative care are poorly understood and can lead to insufficient implementation of HPPC. An incomplete understanding of the scope of HPPC is likely to result in the failure to successfully integrate HPPC. The need for systematic approaches across the whole of organisations and health systems to implementing organisational change is clear.

Note

1 My emphasis.

References

Baum, F. (2008) *The New Public Health* (3rd edn). South Melbourne: Oxford University Press.

Beresford, L. (1993) *The Hospice Handbook*. Boston: Little, Brown and Company.

Buckley, J. (2002) Holism and a health-promoting approach to palliative care. *International Journal of Palliative Nursing*, 8(10), 505–508.

Bunton, R. and MacDonald, G. (2002) *Health Promotion: Disciplines, Diversity and Developments* (2nd edn). London: Routledge.

Byock, I., Norris, K., Curtis, J. R. and Patrick, D. L. (2003) Improving end of life experience and care in the community: a conceptual framework. *Journal of Pain and Symptom Management*, 22(3), 759–772.

Clark, D., Hockley, J. and Ahmedzai, S. (eds) (1997) *New Themes in Palliative Care*. Buckingham: Open University Press.

Connor, S. R. (1998) *Hospice: Practice, Pitfalls and Promise*. Washington: Taylor and Francis.

Department of Health, UK (1995) *A policy framework for commissioning cancer services: report by the export advisory group on cancer to the chief medical officers of England and Wales [The Calman-Hine Report]*. London: Department of Health.

D'Onofrio, C. and Ryndes, T. (2003) The relevance of public health in improving access to end of life care. *The Hastings Center Report*, S30-32.

Douglas, C. (1992) For all the Saints. *The British Medical Journal*, 304, 579.

Elwyn, G. and Rhydderch, M. (2002) Achieving organisational change in primary care: simmer gently for two years. *Preventive Medicine*, 35, 419–421.

Faulkner, M. (1993) Promoting a healthy bereavement. *Journal of Community Nursing*, 18, 23.

Gallagher, R. (2001) Using a trade-show format to educate the public about death and survey public knowledge and needs about issues surrounding death and dying. *Journal of Pain and Symptom Management*, 21(1), 52–58.

Hockley, J. (1997) The evolution of the hospice approach. In D. Clark, J. Hockley and S. Ahmedzai (eds), *New Themes in Palliative Care*. Buckingham: Open University Press.

Howarth, G. (2007) *Death and Dying: a Sociological Introduction*. Cambridge: Polity Press.

Hunt, R. W. and Maddocks, I. (1997) Terminal care in South Australia: historical aspects and equity issues. In D. Clark, J. Hockley and S. Ahmedzai (eds), *New Themes in Palliative Care*. Buckingham: Open University Press.

Kearney, M. (1992) Palliative medicine – just another specialty? *Palliative Medicine*, 6, 39–46.

Kellehear, A. (1999) *Health Promoting Palliative Care*. Oxford: Oxford University Press.

Kellehear, A. (2005) *Compassionate Cities: Public Health and End-of-Life Care*. London: Routledge.

Kellehear, A., Bateman, G. and Rumbold, B. (2003) Practice Guidelines for Health Promoting Palliative Care. Melbourne: La Trobe University.

Lewis, M. (2007) *Medicine and Care of the Dying*. New York: Oxford University Press.

Mor, V., Greer, D. S. and Kastenbaum, R. (1998) *The Hospice Experiment*. Baltimore: Johns Hopkins University Press.

Palliative Care Australia (2005) *A Guide to Palliative Care Service Development – a Population-Based Approach*. Canberra: Palliative Care Australia.

Pegg, B. and Tan, L. (2002) Reducing suffering to improve quality of life through health promotion. *Contemporary Nurse*, 12(1), 22–30.

Rao, J. K., Anderson, L. A. and Smith, S. M. (2002) End-of-life is a public health issue. *American Journal of Preventive Medicine*, 23(3), 215–220.

Rao, J. K., Alongi, J., Anderson, L. A., Jenkins, L., Stokes, G.-A. and Kane, M. (2005) Development of public health priorities for end-of-life care. *American Journal of Preventive Medicine*, 29(5), 453–460.

Richardson, J. (2002) Health promotion in palliative care: the patients' perception of therapeutic interaction with the palliative nurse in the primary care setting. *Journal of Advanced Nursing*, 40(4), 432–440.

Rosenberg, J. P. (1992) *Palliative care in the home – a surprising component of primary health care?* Paper presented at the Primary Health Care: Development and Diversity Conference, Sydney.

Rosenberg, J. P. (2007) *A study of the integration of health promotion principles and practice in palliative care organisations*. PhD thesis. Queensland University of Technology, Brisbane.

Rosenberg, J. P. and Yates, P. M. (2010) Health promotion in palliative care: the case for conceptual congruence. *Critical Public Health*, 20(2), 201–210.

Russell, P. S. and Sander, R. (1998) Health promotion: focus on care of the dying. *International Journal of Palliative Nursing*, 4(6), 266–270.

Salau, S. (2006) *Embedding health promotion philosophy into palliative care*. Paper presented at the Palliative Care Victoria: State Conference, Bendigo.

Scott, J. F. (1992) Palliative care education in Canada: attacking fear and promoting health. *Journal of Palliative Care*, 8(1), 47–53.

Stjaduhar, K. I., Bidgood, D., Norgrove, L., Allan, D. and Waskiewich, S. (2006) Using quality improvement to enhance research readiness in palliative care. *Journal of the National Association for Healthcare Quality*, 28(4), 22–28.

Stjernsward, J. (2007) Palliative care: the Public Health strategy. *Journal of Public Health Policy*, 28(1), 42–55.

vanderPloeg, W. (2001) Health promotion in palliative care: an occupational perspective. *Australian Occupational Therapy Journal*, 48, 45–48.

Weaver, A. W. (2004) Family health promotion during life-threatening illness and at the end of life. In P. J. Bomar (ed.), *Promoting Health In Families* (3rd edn). Philadelphia: Elsevier Inc.

Whitelaw, S., Martin, C., Kerr, A. and Wimbush, E. (2006) An evaluation of the health promoting health service framework: the implementation of a settings based approach with the NHS in Scotland. *Health Promotion International*, 21(2), 136–144.

World Health Organization (1978) *The Declaration of Alma-Ata*. Geneva: WHO.

World Health Organization (1986) *The Ottawa Charter for Health Promotion*. Geneva: WHO.

World Health Organization (1990) *Cancer Pain Relief and Palliative Care [Report No. 804]*. Geneva: WHO.

World Health Organization (1997) *The Jakarta Declaration on Leading Health Promotion into the 21st Century*. Geneva: WHO.

World Health Organization (2006) *The Bangkok Charter for Health Promotion in a Globalised World*. Geneva: WHO.

World Health Organization (2008) Definition of Palliative Care. Available at www.who.int/cancer/palliative/en/ (accessed 18 December 2008).

Zeefe, L. R. (1996) Death Education: Teaching Staff, Patients and Families about the Dying Process. In D. C. Sheehan and W. B. Forman (eds), *Hospice and Palliative Care: Concepts and Practice*. Sudbury: Jones and Bartlett Publishers.

3 Illness trajectories and palliative care

Implications for holistic service provision for all in the last year of life

Scott A. Murray and Peter McLoughlin

Introduction

New theoretical insight into the trajectories of decline in a range of long-term conditions has improved our understanding of people's care and support needs as they approach the end of life. This means that we are now able to make a real difference to the lives of nearly all people in the throes of their final illness, and to the lives of their families (Murray *et al.* 2005). Getting end of life care "right" lies at the heart of what it means to be a civilised society and thus prioritising this area needs no apologies.

Worldwide in 2005 cancer was responsible for a relatively small percentage of deaths (13 per cent), while other long-term conditions caused 47 per cent of all deaths. By 2030 the annual number of deaths around the world is expected to rise from 58 million to 74 million with conditions related to organ failure, and physical and cognitive frailty, responsible for most of this increase. Yet despite these rapid demographic changes, palliative care services typically still cater predominantly for people with cancer. For example, hospices in economically developed countries currently provide 90 per cent of their care to patients with cancer. Moreover, people dying from cancer usually have needs lasting for weeks or months, whereas those dying from organ failure or old age often have unmet needs that extend over many months or years. It is little wonder then that people dying of the "wrong" condition and their carers (whether family, social, or professional) are increasingly frustrated by the major obstacles to accessing appropriate care.

The drive to extend palliative care beyond cancer has so far been hampered by a combination of factors: prognostic uncertainty; funding difficulties; lack of palliative care clinicians with expertise in non-malignant diseases; and a hitherto relatively weak evidence base in relation to appropriate models of care. Although the empirical evidence base remains weak, we do now have a good theoretical understanding of when and how to intervene in a range of conditions. Prognostic uncertainty can and does hinder clinicians, and patients and their families, in thinking and planning ahead. Most patients with heart failure die when they are still expected to live for more than six months. Accurate prognostication is also virtually impossible in people with chronic obstructive pulmonary disease (Glare and Christakis 2004; Lynn and Adamson 2003). But recent work described below may help to identify triggers, or stages, when a palliative approach may be introduced in various illnesses.

Section A: different trajectories for different diseases

A century ago death was typically quite sudden and the leading causes were infections, accidents, and childbirth. Today sudden death is less common, particularly in economically developed societies. Towards the end of life most people acquire serious progressive illness (either one illness, or two or more concurrently). This increasingly interferes with people's ability to continue their usual activities until death. Cardiovascular disease, cancer, and respiratory disorders are the three leading causes of death.

Three distinct "illness trajectories" are described for people with progressive chronic illnesses (World Health Organization 2004; Lunney *et al.* 2003; Murray and Sheikh 2008) (Figure 3.1): a trajectory with steady progression and usually a clear terminal phase, mostly (but not exclusively) cancer; a trajectory with gradual decline, punctuated by episodes of acute deterioration and some recovery, with more sudden, seemingly unexpected death (commonly respiratory and heart failure, for example); and a trajectory with prolonged gradual decline to death (typical of frail elderly people, or people with dementia). These trajectories were first proposed by Lunney *et al.* examining a large quantitative dataset in North America. To understand them better our research group at Edinburgh University has, in a number of studies, used serial qualitative interviews to understand patients' evolving and dynamic experiences and needs in the last

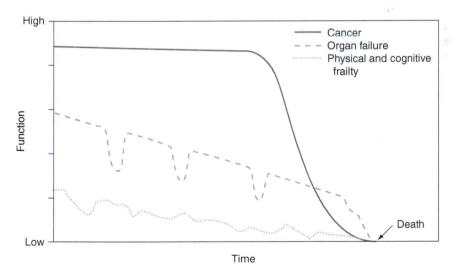

Figure 3.1 The three main trajectories of decline at the end of life (source: Murray and Sheikh 2008).

years of life. We now consider each of these three trajectories in more detail, with illustrations from our research.

Trajectory 1: short period of evident decline

This entails a reasonably predictable decline in physical health over a period of weeks, months, or in some cases years, as is typical in progressive cancer. This course may be punctuated by the positive or negative effects of oncological treatment. Most weight loss, reduction in performance status, and impaired ability for self care occurs in a person's last few months of life. With the trend towards earlier diagnosis and greater openness about discussing prognosis, there is generally time to anticipate palliative needs and plan for end of life care. This trajectory enmeshes well with traditional specialist palliative care services, such as hospices and their associated community palliative care programmes, which historically concentrate on providing comprehensive services in the last weeks or months of life for people with cancer. Resource constraints on hospices and their community teams, plus their association with dying, can limit their availability and acceptability. Case History 1 illustrates this trajectory.

Trajectory 2: long-term limitations with intermittent serious episodes

With conditions such as heart failure and chronic obstructive pulmonary disease, patients are usually ill for many months or years with occasional acute, often severe, exacerbations. Deteriorations are generally associated with admission to hospital and intensive treatment. This clinically intuitive trajectory has sharper dips than are revealed by pooling quantitative data concerning activities of daily living. Each exacerbation may result in death, and although the patient usually survives many such episodes, a gradual deterioration in health and functional status is typical. The timing of death, however, remains uncertain. In one large study, most patients with advanced heart failure died when expected to live for at least a further six months (Lynn and Adamson 2003). Many people with end stage heart failure and chronic obstructive pulmonary disease follow this trajectory, but this may not be the case for some other organ system failures. Case History 2 illustrates this trajectory.

Trajectory 3: prolonged dwindling

People who escape cancer and organ system failure are likely to die at an older age of either brain failure (such as Alzheimer's or other dementia), or generalised frailty of multiple body systems (Murray et al. 2005). This third trajectory is of progressive disability from an already low baseline of cognitive or physical functioning. Such patients may lose weight and functional capacity and then succumb to minor physical events or daily social "hassles" that may in themselves seem trivial but, occurring in combination with declining reserves, can prove fatal. This trajectory may be cut short by death after an acute event such as a fractured neck or femur, or pneumonia, for example. Case History 3 illustrates this trajectory.

Case History 1: a cancer trajectory

CC, a 51-year-old male shop assistant, complained of night sweats, weight loss, and a cough. An x-ray initially suggested a diagnosis of tuberculosis, but a bronchoscopy and a computed tomography scan revealed an inoperable, non-small cell lung cancer. He was offered and accepted palliative chemotherapy when he had already lost considerable weight (too much to allow him to enter a trial). The chemotherapy may have helped control his breathlessness, but he was subsequently admitted owing to vomiting. Looking back, CC expressed regret that he had received chemotherapy:

> *If I had known I was going to be like this . . .*

His wife felt they had lost valuable time together when he had been relatively well.

CC feared a lingering death:

> *I'd love to be able to have a wee turn-off switch, because the way I've felt, there's some poor souls go on for years and years like this, and they never get cured, I wouldn't like to do that.*

CC's wife, in contrast, worried that her husband might die suddenly:

> *When he's sleeping, I keep waking him up, I am so stupid. He'll say, "Will you leave me alone, I'm sleeping." . . . He's not just going to go there and then, I know, but I've got to reassure myself.*

CC died at home three months after diagnosis, cared for by the primary care team, night nurses, and specialist palliative care services. His death had been discussed openly, and nursing, medical, and support staff were available at home.

Case History 2: an organ failure trajectory

Mrs HH, a 65-year-old retired bookkeeper, had been admitted to hospital several times with cardiac failure. She was housebound in her third floor flat and cared for by a devoted husband who accepted little help from social work or community nursing. Previously she had been very outgoing, but was increasingly isolated. Her major concern was that her rapidly deteriorating vision because of diabetes prevented her from completing crosswords, not that she was breathless at rest with heart failure. Her treatment included high dose diuretics and long-term oxygen therapy. She required frequent blood tests. She had raised her prognosis indirectly with her general practitioner, by mentioning to him that her grandson had asked her if she would be around at Christmas. Prognostic uncertainty was a key issue for many heart failure patients and their carers in our study, as illustrated by the following quotations.

> *I take one step forward, then two steps back.*
> (84-year-old, male, retired engineer, living alone, several recent admissions to hospital)

> *I'd like to get better, but I keep getting worse.*
> (72-year old-widow, living alone, psoriasis and arthritis)

> *Things I used to take for granted are now an impossible dream.*
> (75-year-old man, large family nearby, recently celebrated 50th wedding anniversary)

> *There were times last year, when I thought I was going to die.*
> (77-year-old woman, living alone, several periods in hospital with acute breathlessness)

> *It could happen at any time.*
> (Wife of 62-year-old former footballer and taxi driver)

> *I know he won't get better, but don't know how long he's got.*
> (Wife of 77-year-old retired flour mill worker with severe asthma)

Mrs HH died on the way home from a hospital admission due to a nosebleed. She had had these occasionally as she had hypertension and a perforated nasal septum. Attempted resuscitation took place in the ambulance. Her husband later expressed deep regret that this futile attempt had taken place against her, and his, wishes.

Case History 3: a frailty trajectory

Mrs FF, a 92-year-old widow, lives alone in a ground floor flat in central Edinburgh. Bereaved 12 years ago, she is now housebound due to arthritis and general physical frailty. She used to venture out occasionally to the shops but over the years has felt less able and confident, largely because of a fear of falling. She appreciated the chair and walking aids supplied by the occupational therapist as these provided support and a sense of security at home. Since a "little fright" she had before Christmas when her legs gave way, she retires to bed earlier than before. She receives regular visits from friends and the local church and is undemanding of services. Current medications are paracetamol, thyroxin, and bendrofluazide (for hypertension) and an annual influenza vaccine. Mrs LC understands her current trajectory in terms of gradual decline in activities that she is able to do, and she is concerned that she might one day lose her independence or her memory. She has no relatives but is supported by her trust in God, who has "*given me a good while on the planet, and should be sending for me now.*"

Implications for public health and service planning

One size may not fit all

Different models of care will be appropriate for people with different illness trajectories. The typical hospice model of cancer palliative care does not suit people who have a gradual, progressive decline with unpredictable exacerbations. People with non-malignant disease may have more prolonged needs, but these are as pressing as those of people with cancer. Uncertainty about prognosis should not result in these patients, and their families, being relatively neglected by health and social services (World Health Organization 2004; Lunney *et al.* 2003). A strategic overview of the needs of, and services available to, people on the main trajectories may help policies and services to be better conceptualised, formulated, and developed to consider all people with serious chronic illnesses, rather than cancer alone.

Planning care in advance may prevent admissions

Planning care in advance on the basis of these trajectories might help more people to be cared for where and how they would prefer to be, and to die where they would prefer to. For example, currently many frail elderly and patients with dementia are suddenly admitted to hospital to die. Yet, the use of advance care plans and end of life care pathways in nursing homes is proving increasingly effective in preventing such admissions.

Transferable lessons

Models of care for one trajectory may inform another. For example, cancer care can learn from the health promotion paradigm already established in the management of chronic diseases. Improving living while near death in North America, and "health promoting palliative care" in Australia, are two such examples (Kellehear 1999). These have the potential to de-stigmatise death and maximise cancer patients' quality of life right up to death. Conversely, patients with organ failure could benefit from ideas developed in cancer care, such as advance care planning frameworks, and end of life pathways (Gold Standards Framework 2010). There are striking similarities between the burden of symptoms at any time of patients dying of cancer, and those dying of non-malignant cardiorespiratory disease. Hospital palliative care teams, through offering specialist advice and sharing care with other specialists, can improve the care of many non-cancer patients.

Application to health service policy and planning

Implications for service planning have been recognised and built into joint strategic development work undertaken by NHS Lothian (the Health Board with responsibility for health service provision and health improvement in the City

of Edinburgh and East, Mid and West Lothian, covering a total population in
excess of 800,000), the University of Edinburgh Centre for Population Health
Sciences, and the independent hospices in the Lothian area.

The NHS Lothian strategy "Living & Dying Well in Lothian – Lothian's
Palliative Care Strategy 2010–2015" draws upon the conceptual model of
"Trajectories of dying" throughout to help explain how people die, their needs,
demands on health and social care services, and to inform the approach to care
required.

Research into trajectories of dying has provided a new model for strategic
planning. Detailed analysis of mortality data in Lothian confirms that this
model reflects broad patterns of dying in Lothian. Adopting this framework as
an underpinning to health policy and planning helps to overcome a major
hurdle to providing palliative care for all, that is, our concept of how people die.
We have assumed that there is a progressive decline towards death and that, if
we were better at spotting the beginning of this decline, we would be able to
provide palliative care to more people. Trajectory models help both service
planning and care planning to move beyond this. Through the use of trajectories we can better recognise whole patterns of decline (rather than single
points of decline). Consequently we are better able to recognise the multiple
opportunities that exist in the patient pathway to commence and develop a
more supportive and collaborative approach to care. For service planning at
population level, trajectory groupings support a sharper focus for service redesign and opportunities to improve care. A diagrammatic representation of this is
included in Appendix 5.

Clinical implications

Providing appropriate care

Thinking in terms of illness trajectories may help clinicians plan and deliver
appropriate care that integrates active and palliative management, and optimises
quality of life before death. Before the terminal stages of a disease, some health
professionals may allow the reality of the prognosis to remain unconsidered or
unspoken, unwittingly colluding with patients and relatives in fighting death to
the bitter end. Patients often demand palliative oncological treatment even if it
is extremely unlikely to benefit them, and doctors may offer it to maintain hope
as well as to treat disease. An outlook on death, and expectations that are more
acquiescent to reality, may moderate the "technological imperative", preventing
unnecessary admissions to hospital or aggressive treatments. A realistic dialogue
about the illness trajectory between patient, family, and professionals can allow
the option of supportive care, focusing on quality of life and symptom control to
be grasped earlier and more frequently. Figure 3.2 illustrates how the idea that
palliative care is relevant only to the last few weeks of life is being replaced with
the concept that the palliative care approach should be offered increasingly, concurrently, alongside disease modifying or curative treatment.

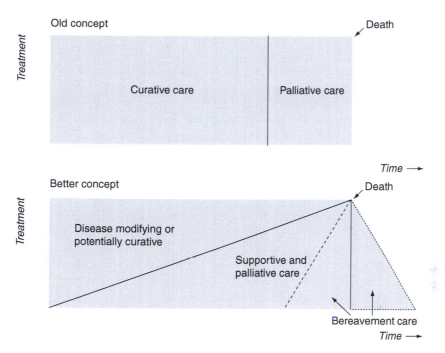

Figure 3.2 When is the palliative care approach indicated? (source: Murray *et al.* 2005).

Trajectories allow practical planning for a "good death"

Dying at home is the expressed wish of around 65 per cent of people at the beginning of the cancer and organ failure trajectories. An appreciation that all trajectories lead to death, but that death may be sudden (particularly in patients following Trajectory 2), makes it evident that advance planning is sensible. Eliciting the "preferred place of care" is now standard in some palliative care frameworks and helps general practitioners plan for care where the patient and family wish. This may increase the likelihood of patients dying in the place of their choice, as was the case for CC (see Case History 1). Sensitive exploration is needed and can allow issues such as resuscitation status to be clarified, and "unfinished business" to be completed for patients on all these trajectories. However, advance directives may be ignored in the heat of the moment. Mrs HH's death had (unusually in people with heart failure) been planned, but an emergency overtook the situation and she received inappropriate resuscitation as documentation was not at hand (Case History 2).

Understanding the likely trajectory may be empowering for patient and carer

If patients and their carers gain a better understanding by considering illness trajectories this may help them feel in greater control of their situation, and empower them to cope with its demands. Had CC (Case History 1), who had lung cancer, been aware of his likely course of decline he might have been less worried about a very protracted death. Similarly, his wife might have been less worried about a sudden death. Both gave clear cues in the research interviews that they were concerned about the possible nature of the death and would have welcomed more information and discussion. But patients must not be simply slotted into a set category without regular review. Individual patients will die at different stages along each trajectory, and the rate of progression may vary. Other diseases or social and family circumstances may intervene, so that priorities and needs change.

Summary points from Section A

- Three typical illness trajectories have been described for patients with progressive chronic illness: cancer, organ failure, and the frail elderly or dementia trajectory.
- Different models of care will be appropriate for people with different illness trajectories, and service redesign will be required to establish services that best fit the non-cancer trajectories.
- Being aware of these trajectories may help clinicians plan timely appropriate care, and take on board at an earlier stage that progressive deterioration and death are inevitable, and help patients and carers cope with their situation.

Section B: multidimensional illness trajectories

Although physical needs tend to occupy centre stage in medicine, it is important to be aware that people with progressive malignant and non-malignant illnesses have multidimensional needs (McClain and Rosenfeld 2003). The World Health Organization (WHO) states that palliative care seeks to prevent and relieve suffering through early identification, assessment, and management of pain and other problems, whether physical, psychosocial, or spiritual (2004). Quality of life, and of death, is modified by all domains of personhood (Cassell 1991). Saunders has described the multidimensional suffering of "total pain" as a lack of personal integrity and inner peace (Saunders 1996). In reality, social needs may be pressing but neglected (Clausen *et al.* 2005). From the moment someone learns that cure is not possible, that person sees himself or herself differently and is perceived differently by those around them (Sheldon 2003).

Psychological distress, both anxiety and depression, are well documented in advanced illness, and frequently under diagnosed. The existential or spiritual domain is another determinant of quality of life that can influence treatment decisions. Belief systems and spirituality (defined as existential rather than religious belief) are important to 70–80 per cent of the general population in the UK, and to 90 per cent of elderly patients in the United States. In cancer and palliative care, spiritual distress is associated with psychosocial needs, communication issues, death anxiety, and despair. Near the end of life, issues relating to the meaning and purpose of life have been found to be more important than physical symptoms, physical wellbeing, or support, and may be responsive to palliative care interventions (Puchalski *et al.* 2003).

We define the social domain as relating to the carer's ability to network and generally socialise, the psychological domain as relating to their mental wellbeing, including anxiety and depression, and spiritual need as:

> The needs and expectations which humans have to find meaning, purpose and value in their life. Such needs can be specifically religious, but even people who have no religious faith or are not members of an organized religion have belief systems that give their lives meaning and purpose.
>
> (Institute of Medicine 1997)

Our research group explored whether there were common trajectories of social, psychological, and spiritual wellbeing by synthesising data from two longitudinal, qualitative, in-depth interview studies of people with lung cancer and heart failure which they had previously carried out. We noted when patients tended to have distress in these different dimensions, and mapped out such patterns (Murray *et al.* 2007). We illustrate this in the text below using some of the quotations.

Lung cancer trajectories

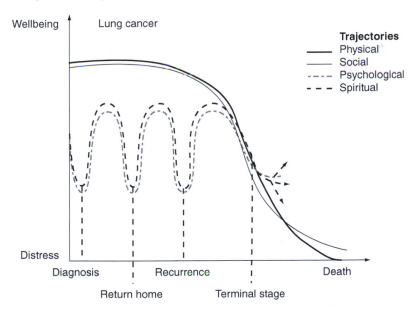

Figure 3.3 Lung cancer: physical, social, psychological and spiritual trajectories.

Social needs

As physical limitations increased, either from the illness itself or from treatment side effects, there was often a parallel decline in social wellbeing. Relationships with friends could be uneasy due to the stigma of a cancer diagnosis. *"There's old friends won't even take a cup of tea with me now I've got cancer"* Mrs LR. Many patients spoke of feeling increasingly useless, dependent, and sometimes excluded from their usual family and social roles by well meaning relatives. Towards the terminal phase, people's social world tended to shrink down to family, and then just self.

Psychological needs

Patients with advanced lung cancer tended to experience uncertainty and emotional distress at four key stages or transitions: diagnosis, discharge after treatment, disease progression, and the terminal stages (Figure 3.3). These caused four troughs in the graph of typical psychological wellbeing. Initially, while waiting for test results and the start of treatment, patients were highly anxious, emotionally distressed, and perceived a lack of support. For those who heard at diagnosis that the cancer was both inoperable and incurable, this was especially devastating.

> *Well, I got the results back that afternoon and he said "I'm afraid it's terminal." I got such a shock it was like as if he was talking about someone else because other than that I was feeling fine. We were absolutely gob-smacked.*
>
> Mrs LQ

Once treatment started, patients felt more supported through contact with various staff, and the atmosphere of hope that the activity of treatment instigated. *"The treatments have helped as well. Great nurses and departments, eh, specialists. They're so caring. The oncology people, I mean, they get to know their patients so well, you know."* Mr LK

After treatment there was often, but not always, a recurrence of psychological distress, especially if there was little contact with hospital or primary care. Many patients struggled to return to their old life, finding it hard to cope with changes in body image and their new identity as a cancer patient. *"It was like a black hole."* Ms LP

At relapse, or when there was disease progression, patients were challenged again. For some, engaging in a battle to defeat the cancer appeared to give them a sense of purpose and enabled them to cope. Others reflected on the progressive losses experienced throughout their illness. *"I feel useless. When the quality has gone, life isn't your own."* Mrs LU

In the terminal phase, some patients routinely contacted health services for reassurance, often describing physical symptoms to legitimize the call. An overwhelming sense of uncertainty, with frequent panic attacks, prevented one patient from dying at home. *"You don't know what is going to happen to you, fear is the worst thing."* Mrs LI

Spiritual needs

For patients with lung cancer, spiritual distress and questioning tended to occur at the same four points of transition as psychological distress (Figure 3.1). At diagnosis, patients came face to face with the prospect of suffering and death. They had difficulties of explaining their emptiness and searching: *"Maybe this is God turning 'round and saying 'I'm going to get you back,' because I've not always been a lily-white guy."* Mr LC

Returning home at the end of inpatient treatment, many patients struggled to return to their old life, and spoke of an altered sense of self and a questioning of self-worth and their value to others. At disease progression, some people wondered what they had achieved in their lives and what needed to be done before death. Some patients, perceiving that they had no future, felt that their life in the present was pointless. In the terminal phase, an acceptance of death was sometimes apparent. Some worried if they had been good enough during their life, if there was an afterlife, and feared to die. Others felt confident in their faith, knowing that death was a transition rather than the end. *"I'll say, 'God just let me die tonight,' there must be something that's better than this."* Mr LV

Heart failure trajectory

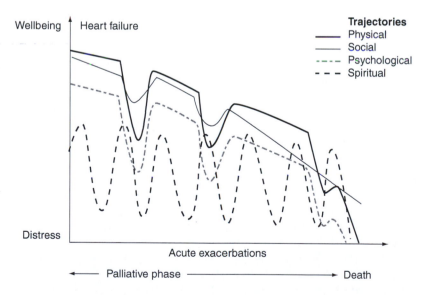

Figure 3.4 Heart failure: physical, social, psychological and spiritual trajectories (Murray *et al.* 2007).

Social needs

As physical decline gradually progressed, with exacerbations sometimes necessitating hospital admission, there was a parallel shrinking social world. In HH's case, planning to go out was fraught due to the fluctuations in the illness and having to find a toilet frequently due to the diuretic medication. The patient's sense of imprisonment was exacerbated by relatives who unintentionally treated them as the "invalid", confirming their loss of independence and previous identity. Social support was less available than for people with cancer, although most preferred to be at home.

Psychological needs

Psychological wellbeing appeared to mirror the physical and social trajectories. Acute anxiety often accompanied sudden physical exacerbations. *"I slipped down the bed and oh, panic attacks I got, and had to sit up. I couldn't get my breath. You can't actually tell people."* Mr HQ

Fluctuating but progressive physical debility and increasing social isolation generally caused frustration and low mood. However, some patients did adopt a resilient, almost stoical approach. *"It's going to be what it's going to be the rest of time I've got left I am just taking each day as it comes."* Mrs HW

Spiritual needs

Spiritual wellbeing in people with heart failure gradually decreased, although sometimes varied throughout the trajectory. This reflected a progressive loss of identity and growing dependence. Displacement within the family echoed a sense of displacement within a greater scheme of things, and left patients questioning their value and place in the world. As their illness incapacitated them, patients searched for meaning. Patients who felt valued and affirmed described being more able to come to terms with their life, and retain a sense of worth and meaning. Illness and suffering was sometimes associated with positive aspects, such as love, hope, trust, forgiveness. While some were supported and comforted by their religious beliefs, others wondered about judgment or divine indifference. *"Where is God in all this, has God forsaken me?"* Mr HU

As they sensed the imminence of death, some heart failure patients, like those with lung cancer, asked more explicit questions. *"Is it real, is there life after death, where am I going?"* *"What happens if I am wrong and there is something after all?"* Mrs HV

In summary, in lung cancer, the physical and social trajectories appeared interlinked. People tended to describe themselves as having more psychological and spiritual distress at four specific transitions. In advanced heart failure, the physical and both the social and psychological decline appeared interlinked, following the pattern of physical deterioration. Spiritual distress fluctuated more and was modulated by various other influences, including a perceived lack of understanding of these issues by health professionals.

Implications for public health and service planning

Raising social issues may help more people die where they wish. In the economically developed world, dying at home is the express wish of around 65 per cent of people at the beginning of both cancer and organ failure trajectories, although few achieve this (Gomes and Higginson 2006). In the United States and the UK, only around 20 per cent die at home, whereas in Eire, 60 per cent do so. Eliciting social factors, including the "preferred place of care", now routine in the UK Gold Standards Framework (2010), greatly helps advance planning, which is central to effective care. Primary care teams report more people dying in their preferred place when these social aspects are broached. The Liverpool End of Life Care Pathway promotes the proactive identification of multidimensional needs in the last days of life. Dealing with social and practical issues is likely to contribute to a decrease in emergency admissions, including the many due to carer distress.

Spiritual assessment and care should be part of care. Many patients have spiritual issues from the diagnosis of a life-threatening cancer or chronic condition, not just at the very end of life. A patient-centred approach, supporting people in their own worldview, and providing openings for expression of fear, doubt, and anxiety may help patients in their search for meaning, and prevent spiritual concerns amounting to disabling distress. This multidimensional approach is ideally suited to all patients with serious medical conditions; it should not be confined to only those actively dying.

Application to health service policy and planning

The strategic principles for service redesign in palliative and end of life care in NHS Lothian include "*early holistic assessment and intervention; patients and carers involved and engaged with their care; and delivering care planning which involves people, establishing and working towards achieving their preference for place of care and place of death.*" These are key components which are being increasingly reflected in the delivery of anticipatory and advance care planning in NHS Lothian. This framework of four interlinked trajectories maps well to a range of patient focused anticipatory care domains of work in development across NHS Lothian. Recognising the interlinkage of physical, social, psychological and spiritual trajectories, and the common points in the patient pathway where specific intervention opportunities exist for patients and their carers alike (at diagnosis, upon discharge post treatment, upon disease progression or recurrence, and close to death) supports the further development of holistic and personalised care provision.

Working in partnership with the primary palliative care research programme in Edinburgh by developing and adapting the research programme will assist in both evaluating NHS Lothian strategy implementation and developing plans for service redesign in palliative and end of life care.

Clinical implications

Care planning must be four-dimensional. Understanding and considering typical trajectories may help professionals anticipate when, and in which dimension, an individual patient is likely to be distressed. Equipped with this, they are in a better position to plan care proactively. Furthermore, some patients attempt to gain control over their illness by acquiring knowledge about how it is likely to progress. Explanation about when practical, emotional, and existential issues might be expected to occur, and the services available should they do so, could empower patients and their carers.

Clinicians should adopt their own simple but comprehensive assessment tool for all their patients who might die soon. We are not suggesting that health professionals should take the responsibility for dealing with all dimensions of need. Rather, that they should be able to recognise unmet needs that are causing significant distress, and provide adequate information and support, or refer to other social and spiritual care providers, if the patient wishes. A holistic approach considering each dimension of need may moderate the current "technological imperative", with care focused on physical interventions to preserve or prolong life. A realistic dialogue acknowledging the different trajectories and dimensions of needs with the patient, family, and professionals can allow the option of supportive care, focusing on quality of life and symptom control, to be adopted earlier and more frequently (Murray *et al.* 2005).

Summary points from Section B

- In lung cancer, the social trajectory mirrored physical decline, while psychological and spiritual wellbeing decreased together at four key transitions: diagnosis, discharge after treatment, disease progression, and the terminal stage.
- In advanced heart failure, both social and psychological decline tended to track the physical decline, while spiritual distress exhibited background fluctuations.
- High quality holistic end of life care should encompass all these dimensions.
- An appreciation of common patterns of not only physical but social, psychological, and spiritual wellbeing and decline may assist clinicians as they discuss the likely course of events with patients and carers. It may also help with attempts to minimise distress as the disease progresses.

Section C: multidimensional trajectories in family carers of people with cancer

Since 1995 UK health policies have acknowledged that informal carers of patients with cancer have views and preferences that should be considered alongside those of patients, and that services should support carers as well as patients (Department of Health 2008). Cancer is recognised increasingly as affecting all the family, with psychological distress reverberating substantially throughout the nuclear family and perhaps beyond. Psychological distress is the most researched aspect of quality of life in carers. Most studies, including a recent systematic review and meta-analysis, suggest a positive association between patients' and carers' psychological distress (Kissanne *et al.* 1994). The mental health of carers of people with lung cancer is thought to be more at risk as the illness progresses, particularly when patients have advanced disease. Other factors that might also affect the level of, and relation between, psychological distress experienced by patients and their carers have received insufficient attention. Evidence is beginning to accumulate on the detrimental impact of cancer on the physical health and spiritual wellbeing of family caregivers (Kim and Given 2008).

Building on our previous work in this area, (Murray *et al.* 2009; Kendall *et al.* 2009), we explored if typical trajectories existed in carers by considering and plotting at what stage in the illness pathway we had carried out each interview, and what dimensions of distress in carers were vocalised by the patients and carers at these time points. Such secondary analysis of data produced by qualitative research is an established approach to the generation of new knowledge in the discipline of health care. Again these are illustrated below by the use of quotations.

Trajectories of physical, social, psychological and spiritual wellbeing

Archetypal trajectories of social, psychological, and spiritual wellbeing were found in carers. The multidimensional experience of distress suffered by their loved ones was reflected in their own suffering, and being most pronounced for psychological and spiritual distress (Murray *et al.* 2010). As carers' multidimensional needs were dynamic and variable, quotations and graphic representations are presented to highlight and explain the patterns that emerged (Figure 3.5).

Physical wellbeing

Data on the health status of carers were relatively sparse, but where present these data suggested that carers' own physical health might suffer. This could compromise their capacity to care; some also felt exhausted and that they were sharing the illness, especially as time went on and death approached.

Social wellbeing

As patients became progressively unwell the carer often felt less and less able to leave them alone. This often meant restricting their own normal social contacts, hobbies, work, and even holidays. Other family members might also be more reluctant to visit, leaving the carer feeling physically and socially isolated, as if they too had moved into a life centred on illness and were in a parallel

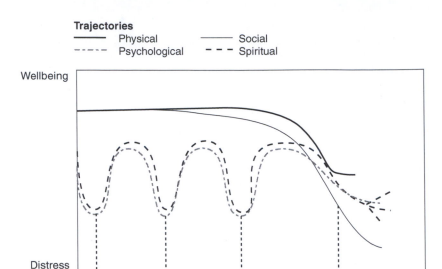

Figure 3.5 Trajectories of physical, social, and psychological and spiritual wellbeing in family carers of patients with lung cancer, from diagnosis to death (source: Murray *et al.* 2010).

world with the patient. This diminishment of existing social contacts added to the sense of loss and isolation when bereaved.

Psychological wellbeing

Carers, like patients, often felt they were on an emotional rollercoaster experiencing peaks and troughs at key times of stress and uncertainty in the cancer trajectory. The time of diagnosis was surrounded with particularly acute anxiety: "*It's just like being hit by a train, isn't it? . . . It's just like, you, you just hear the word . . . [a month on] you still cannae take it in.*"

At home after initial treatment, trying to communicate in itself was distressing, and the carer could feel increasingly worn down and under pressure: "*Tired of it! Yes, you get fed up . . . I think we do feel that the pressure is getting to us really. It has been hard, it's not easy for us to say that. . . . But yes, it is difficult.*"

When the disease recurred carers might empathise with the worry the patients had at that stage, but sometimes had to deal with difficult behaviour, along with their own concerns that their partner might suddenly die: "*He went through a phase where he [husband] was really aggressive and very moody and he was terrible—it just drives me crazy.*"

At the terminal stage, one carer sat up at night worried that her husband might die soon.

Spiritual wellbeing

Spiritually distressed carers also often considered why the illness had appeared. With the patient back home, some carers tried intellectually to accept the diagnosis and prognosis but were still emotionally upset:

> *Well, it's just something I've got to accept. Nothing I can do about it, so what's the use of worrying about it? I would have said just enjoy each day as it comes, but that's just it, with all this, you cannae enjoy yourself.*

One carer, when learning that the patient's cancer was advanced, found solace in retreating to the bathroom to pray, whereas another was confused that God did not seem to be present in their suffering.

At the terminal stage, another carer felt her hopes would be dashed if her husband left her house, their sanctuary: *"All my hope will have gone if he is to go into the hospice. I really, really don't want him to die in there"*.

Implications for public health and service planning

Our work suggests that, in addition to the recognised bereavement phase, the key time points to focus psychological and existential support for carers are at diagnosis, at home after initial treatment, at recurrence, and in the terminal stage. As these key time points are the same for patients, the needs of patients and carers should be dealt with in parallel. Family carers witness and share much of the illness experience of the dying person, albeit in their own distinct ways. The multidimensional experience of distress suffered by patients with lung cancer tends to be mirrored by their carers. The patterns that we describe resonate with the turbulent experiences of patients, these being shaped to an extent by the nature of the illness and the care available. The fact that distress in carers can be most acute at around the time of diagnosis of a life-threatening illness leads us to suggest that initiative to identify and support family carers should be done early in the course of the illness, rather than when the patient needs physical support at the end of life. General practitioners are currently encouraged through the UK Quality and Outcome framework to identify carers: this should be done earlier rather than later.

Although most medical conditions have "typical presentations", cases present and evolve in various ways. Illnesses can only be experienced in a family or community context, which can be highly individual and change according to circumstances, including care setting. Thus there is a danger of stereotyping on the basis of archetypal trajectories, and further work is needed to explore these, and other patterns or sub-trajectories, in patients and carers. Carers can, and may be encouraged to, draw on resources within themselves or from others to moderate the distress that might otherwise occur. The predictive value at the level of the individual may be limited, but there are, nonetheless, clear policy implications for providing adequate services for carers so that services are configured to be person centred and timely.

Clinical implications

Proactive support and management should be targeted at critical stages to minimise the risk of predictable distress in carers. It may also be empowering for
carers to know that it is common to feel stressed and in need of support at
certain times. Clinical implications may be especially relevant in primary care,
where the patient and carer are often both supported by the same clinicians. A
previous study of carers of patients with lung cancer found that the main component of emotional support for them was having someone to listen and talk to.
We suggest this support should be available not just in the terminal phase or in
bereavement but at the four key transitions: at diagnosis, at home after treatment, at recurrence, and in the terminal stage. These findings are also likely to
apply to carers of people affected by other cancers that are characterised by rapid
decline.

Summary points from Section C

- Family caregivers may experience typical patterns of wellbeing and distress
  in parallel with patients.
- Psychosocial and existential support for patients with lung cancer and their
  family carers should be offered not just in the terminal phase or in bereavement but at four key transitions: at diagnosis, at home after initial treatment, at recurrence, and in the terminal stage.

Conclusion

Palliative and end of life care must be radically transformed so that people dying
of all illnesses and their carers get reliable and good quality equitable care
(Garber and Leadbeater 2010). The changes needed include both quality
improvements and also radical redesign of care for people at the end of
life. People on the organ failure and frailty trajectories would especially benefit
from redesigned or reinvented services. Further changes needed include
extending the palliative approach to institutions such as care homes, and
promoting a public discourse and community involvement in palliative and
end of life care (Kellehear 1999). Figure 3.6 is a useful framework to consider
how such developments can be conceptualised within four groups: either sustaining or disruptive innovations, either inside or outside palliative care
services.

	Inside	Outside
Sustaining innovation	Improve	Combine
Disruptive innovation	Reinvent	Transform

Figure 3.6 Four categories of end of life developments.

Endnote

In Hippocrates' day, the physician who could foretell the course of the illness was most highly esteemed, even if he could not alter it (Cassell 1991). Nowadays we can cure some diseases and manage others effectively. Where we cannot alter the course of events, we must at least (when the patient so wishes) predict sensitively and together plan holistic care, for better or for worse.

Facilitating a good death should be recognised as a core clinical proficiency, as basic as diagnosis and treatment. Death should be managed properly, integrating technical expertise with a humanistic and ethical orientation. We also need services configured to routinely care well for all patients who are sick enough to die, and we need education that keeps alive our humanity and sense of vocation. This is an enormous public health challenge in politicised, market driven health care models but one that will make an important difference to those most in need.

Acknowledgements

The authors would like to thank members of the Primary Palliative Care Research Group, University of Edinburgh, for carrying out the research described. Thanks are also due to members of the Lothian Palliative Care Managed Clinical Network, and professional and public contributors from across Lothian, for their contribution to strategy development work in NHS Lothian. We thank the Chief Scientist Office of the Scottish Executive, Lothian Health and Macmillan Cancer Support for funding the research studies.

References

Cassell, E. 1991. *The nature of suffering.* New York: Oxford University Press.
Clausen, H., Kendall, M., Murray, S.A., Worth, A., Boyd, K. and Benton, F. 2005. Would palliative care patients benefit from social workers retaining the traditional "casework" role rather than working as care managers? A prospective serial qualitative interview study. *British Journal of Social Work,* 35: 277–85.
Department of Health. 2008. *End of life strategy.* Stationery Office.
Garber, J. and Leadbeater, C. 2010. *Dying for change.* Demos, London.
Glare, P.A. and Christakis, N.A. 2004. *Predicting survival in patients with advanced disease.* In Doyle, D., Hanks, G., Cherny, N. and Calman, K., eds. *Oxford Textbook of Palliative Medicine.* Oxford: Oxford University Press.
Gomes, B. and Higginson, I.J. 2006. Factors influencing death at home in terminally ill patients with cancer: systematic review. *BMJ,* 332: 515–18.
Hockley, J., Watson, J., Oxenham, D. and Murray, S.A. 2010. The integrated implementation of two end of life care tools in nursing care homes in the UK: an in-depth evaluation. *Palliative Medicine,* 24: 828. DOI: 10.1177/0269216310373162.
Institute of Medicine. 1997. *Approaching death. Improving care at the end of life.* Washington, DC: National Academy Press.

Kellehear, A. 1999. *Health Promoting Palliative Care*. Melbourne: Oxford University Press.

Kendall, M., Murray, S.A., Carduff, E., Worth, A., Harris, F., Lloyd, A., *et al.* 2009. Use of multi-perspective qualitative interviews to understand patients' and carers' beliefs, experiences and needs. *BMJ*, 339: b4122.

Kim, Y. and Given, B.A. 2008. Quality of life of family caregivers of cancer survivors across the trajectory of the illness. *Cancer*, 112: 2556–68.

Kissanne, D., Bloch, S., Burns, W.I., Mackenzie, D. and Posterino, M. 1994. Psychological morbidity in the families of patients with cancer. *Psychooncology*, 3: 47–56.

Lunney, J.R., Lynn, J., Foley, D.S., Lipson, S. and Guralnik, J.M. 2003. Patterns of functional decline at the end of life. *JAMA*, 289: 2387–92.

Lynn, J. and Adamson, D.M. 2003. *Living well at the end of life. Adapting health care to serious chronic illness in old age*. Washington: Rand Health.

McClain, C.S. and Rosenfeld, B. 2003. Effect of spiritual well-being on end-of-life in terminally-ill cancer patients. *Lancet*, 361: 1603–7.

Murray, S.A. and Sheikh, A. 2008. Care for all at the end of life. *BMJ*, 336: 958–9.

Murray, S.A., Kendall, M., Boyd, K. and Sheikh, A. 2005. Illness trajectories and palliative care. Clinical Review. *BMJ*, 330: 1007–11.

Murray, S.A., Kendall, M., Boyd, K., Grant, E., Highet, G. and Sheikh, A. 2010. Archetypal trajectories of social, psychological and spiritual wellbeing in family caregivers: secondary analyses of serial qualitative interviews with people with lung cancer and their family caregivers from diagnosis to death. *BMJ*, 304: c2581.

Murray, S., Kendall, M., Carduff, E., Worth, A., Harris, F., Lloyd, A., *et al.* 2009. Use of serial qualitative interviews to understand patients' evolving experiences and needs. *BMJ*, 3009: b3702.

Murray, S.A., Kendall, M., Grant, E., Boyd, K., Barclay, S. and Sheikh, A. 2007. Patterns of social, psychological and spiritual decline towards the end of life in lung cancer and heart failure. *Journal of Pain and Symptom Management*, 34: 393–402.

Puchalski, C.M., Kilpatrick, S.D., McCullough, M.E. and Larson, D. 2003. A systematic review of spiritual and religious variables in Palliative Medicine, *American Journal of Hospice Care*, 1: 7–13.

Saunders, C. 1996. Into the valley of the shadow of death: a personal therapeutic journey. *BMJ*, 313: 1599–1601.

Sheldon, F. 2003. Social impact of advanced metastatic cancer. In Lloyd-Williams, M. ed. Psychosocial issues in palliative care. Oxford: Oxford University Press: 35–48.

The Gold Standards Framework. 2010. A programme for community palliative care. Available from www.goldstandardsframework.nhs.uk.

World Health Organization. 2004. *Palliative care: the solid facts*.

Additional educational resources

For managers and clinicians

Lynn, J. 2004. *Sick to death and not going to take it any more. Reforming health care for the last years of life*. Berkeley, CA: University of California Press.

Lynn, J., Schuster, J.L. and Kabcenell, A. 2000. *Improving care for the end of life: a sourcebook for health care managers and clinicians*. New York: Oxford University Press.

Macmillan Cancer Relief. 2004. *Our principles of patient-centred care*. Available at www.professionalresources.org.uk/Macmillan.

NHS Modernisation Agency. 2004. *Liverpool care pathway. Promoting best practice for the care of the dying. User Guide*. Liverpool: NHS Modernisation Agency. Available at www.lcp-mariecurie.org.uk.

Thomas, K. 2003. *Caring for the dying at home. Companions on a journey*. Oxford: Radcliffe Medical Press.

World Health Organization Europe. 2004 *Better palliative care for older people*. Copenhagen: WHO.

4 Public health approaches to palliative care in Australia

Bruce Rumbold

Introduction

In Australia, as in most other places, palliative care had its origins in the grass-roots community hospice movement. This movement took shape and gathered momentum as local communities in various parts of the world responded to the demonstration project Cicely Saunders set up at St Christopher's Hospice in London in 1967. The St Christopher's hospice philosophy asserted that it is possible to pursue health even in the final days of life: the experience of dying was seen as giving dying people an opportunity to 'make their journey toward their ultimate goals' (Saunders 1996, p. 319). For hospice practitioners symptom control was a means to a wider end: physical comfort should allow dying people and their families to attend to relationships, life review, and spiritual nurture.

Throughout the 1970s in the UK and the USA, and the 1980s in Australia, community networks established and promoted hospice care as a preferred alternative to death in the hospital. By the 1990s, however, the momentum was dissipating, funding pressures were growing, and the community-based hospice programs began to seek a place within mainstream funded health systems. In Australia at least mainstreaming shifted the holistic hospice approach towards clinical care, a more-or-less inevitable consequence of participating in the funding and accountability structures of the health services. Mainstreaming also weakened hospices' alignment with their local communities by amalgamating local hospice groups to increase the catchment areas of the resultant new palliative care services (Rumbold 1998). Certainly mainstreaming resulted in sustainability and improved access to palliative care; but it has also tended to emphasise clinical care, placing allied health in a support role.

Health promoting palliative care

Health promoting approaches were introduced to Australian palliative care by Allan Kellehear, conceptually through his book *Health Promoting Palliative Care* (1999a) and practically by his successful lobbying to obtain government funding to establish a palliative care unit in the School of Public Health, La Trobe University (Kellehear 1999b). Health Promoting Palliative Care (HPPC) was developed as both a response to and a remedy for the contemporary developments in palliative care noted above. It sought to restore to palliative care the holistic perspective of the hospice movement, using the new public health as a framework (see Chapter 1).

Early health promoting strategies initiated by the La Trobe University Palliative Care Unit included conducting health promotion groups with people living with life-limiting illness, and providing education for palliative care providers in health promoting approaches (Kellehear 1999b). The response of practitioners and services to the education program formed a basis for implementation and policy development.

The focus of HPPC was upon reformation of mainstream palliative care practice. A further development, similarly informed by public health thinking, took shape over the first few years of the Unit's life as a response to policy and practice issues arising as services sought to implement HPPC and explore the community development aspects of a public health approach. This expanded model, published as *Compassionate Cities* (Kellehear 2005), brought palliative care practice into dialogue with the healthy settings movement (World Health Organization 1980), in particular the Healthy Cities programme.

Reception of the HPPC model

Initial reception of the model was mixed, best exemplified by the fact that the La Trobe University Palliative Care Unit was funded initially by ministerial decree against the advice of the palliative care section of the Victorian Government Department of Human Services. In the field, responses also varied. Some practitioners were enthusiastic, seeing the model as tackling problems of which they were aware, but which they felt relatively powerless to address. Others were dismissive, suggesting from a superficial reading of HPPC that their services were already doing health promotion, by which they usually meant marketing the service. In response to this, the Unit published practice guidelines (Kellehear *et al.* 2005), designed to spell out what a health promoting approach might involve. Yet others saw the ideas as a good thing, but considered that any such initiatives should be funded from outside the (clinically-focused) palliative care budget: HPPC was seen not to be 'core business'.

Nevertheless, as word spread, local champions emerged to implement HPPC approaches in their own services and regions. The interest generated by the HPPC model, and by projects based upon it, resulted in growing acceptance at the national level of the legitimacy of public health approaches in palliative care, and the need for services to see this as an aspect of practice. By 2003 the national peak body, Palliative Care Australia, in its Service Provision Planning Guide (PCA 2003, p. 13) asked that all services involve themselves in at least one of:

- Community development
- Community education

- Prevention strategies aimed at reducing social morbidity
- Social policy, practices and advice.

This policy affirmation provided support to various local projects that were already taking shape, and also led to the federal Department of Health and Ageing 'Caring Communities' funding round (Quinsey *et al.* 2006; Williams *et al.* 2006) that generated further initiatives. Several key examples based upon HPPC principles are worthy of mention. (These are selected in part because further information on each project is available in published chapters or articles, cited at the end of each summary.)

Schools-based death education program

The Division of Palliative Care at the Mater Misericordiae Hospital, Newcastle, provides both in-patient and community-based palliative care services to the Hunter Region of New South Wales. A series of café conversations (www. theworldcafe.com) was initiated by the Division as a strategy for facilitating community discussion of end of life issues. From these general conversations the idea of providing some form of death education in secondary schools emerged. Discussions were then held with school authorities and, in due course, a café conversation approach was used with teachers as a way of exploring their experiences of dealing with death in the classroom. These conversations identified a range of issues, with priority given to a need for knowing what to say to those affected by bereavement. Accordingly, workshops on bereavement, with a specific focus on communication, were provided to teachers by Division staff. Feedback on these linked programs underlined participants' sense of discovery of their own capacity to talk openly about death, with the café conversations identified as instrumental in this (Kellehear and O'Connor 2008).

Building rural community capacity through volunteering

The Hume Regional Palliative Care Service, in north-west Victoria, generated a remarkable series of initiatives throughout the region with the assistance of funding from the Caring Communities program. The project began with interested palliative care staff and volunteers, but before long others beyond the palliative care arena became involved. A core group of 'health promotion champions' formed a Health Promotion Resource Team. Their task was to encourage community interest in end of life concerns, to mentor community services and groups that expressed an interest, and to elicit, evaluate and support through seed funding local projects that utilised a health promoting approach to a particular end of life issue. As in Newcastle, café conversations were used initially to raise general community awareness, and from there local project ideas germinated. Schools, aged care facilities, community health services, service clubs, faith communities, local government and neighborhood houses were among the community services and groups that formed project partnerships with their local palliative care service. One of the notable features of this program was just how much community involvement could be catalysed with some strategic advice and modest seeding grants (Kellehear and Young 2007; Salau *et al.* 2007). In the course of the Caring Communities Program, the Hume Region developed a simple guidance tool, 'The Big Seven', for designing and assessing health promoting project proposals (Kellehear and Young 2007).

Integrating HPPC in a palliative care service

Early interest in HPPC in Queensland was expressed through Palliative Care Queensland's appointment of a health promotion worker to raise community awareness of health promoting approaches (Colen 2004). This was background to the substantive work undertaken by John Rosenberg in his doctoral project on implementing HPPC in a specialist palliative care service in Brisbane. By capturing multiple perspectives of the change process, he identified as key themes the central importance of a perceived conceptual congruence between health promotion and palliative care, and the need for an intentional and systematic approach to organisational change if the transition was to be effective and beneficial for all involved (Rosenberg 2007; Rosenberg and Yates 2010; see also Chapter 2).

Workplace support

Building upon the HPPC model's interest in developing social support, Palliative Care Victoria, also funded by a Caring Communities Grant, undertook a project to develop a best practice model of support in the workplace for people with a life-threatening illness and employed carers. Respondents to the study included not only carers and those living with illness, but also employers/managers and work colleagues. A profile of needs was drawn up, and strategies for economic, emotional, information and appraisal support identified (Bottomley and Tehan 2005).

Reception of HPPC: expanding horizons

The HPPC model can be seen as an intervention in the field of Australian palliative care. Its intention was to restore a balance to practice by calling attention to social and spiritual aspects in particular that were neglected through the process of mainstreaming. In this sense it offered a radical critique of the field. The consequences of the critique included not only the adoption in some quarters of health promoting approaches, but also the appearance of complementary or alternative approaches. Needs-based population health models have become a principal alternative for developing palliative care policy that takes account of community needs. This approach contains aspects of a public health perspective, but focuses upon a professionalised health service response more than a community response in general.

At the same time that the Palliative Care Australia Service Planning Guide with its public health practice requirements was published, two further initiatives were taking shape. The first was a comprehensive project developing a palliative approach in relation to residential aged care (Australian Government Department of Health and Ageing 2004). The second was a needs-based population health approach, foreshadowed in 2004 (Currow *et al.* 2004) and published as policy a little over a year later by Palliative Care Australia (PCA, 2005). Both initiatives respond to the increasing acceptance of palliative care as a health service: successful community and public education means more people expect access to this type of care.

The palliative approach aims to improve the quality of life for people with a life-limiting illness, and their families, through early identification, assessment and treatment of physical, psychological, socio-cultural and spiritual needs (Kristjanson *et al.* 2003). As such it is not limited to the end stages of an illness, but provides active support and care. It is, as noted in the resultant *Guidelines* themselves, 'an important contribution to Palliative Care Australia's mission to improve palliative care options available to ALL Australians through advocacy and setting high standards for practice, policy, research, and service and community development' (Australian Government Department of Health and Ageing 2004, p. xi).

The needs-based framework (PCA 2005) articulates specialist palliative care services with wider health services and resources offered to people with life-limiting illness: that is, it takes a further step toward introducing palliative care practice to the broad spectrum of end of life needs in Australian society. One significant strategy emanating from this approach provides training for primary care practitioners, through the Program of Experience in the Palliative Approach (PEPA), in the fundamental philosophy and skills of palliative care. It is hoped that the resultant increase in primary practice expertise will lead to more appropriate referrals to specialist services, and that the specialist services in turn will develop consultation with and training for primary care practitioners alongside their delivery of services to those with complex palliative needs. This is represented diagrammatically in Figure 4.1.

Group A, the largest group in Figure 4.1, have their needs met by primary care givers without recourse to either consultancy from or referral to specialist palliative care services. Group B is made up of those who, from time to time, need consultancy and advice from specialist palliative care practitioners, but whose care is largely undertaken by primary care practitioners. Group C have complex needs that require individualised care plans devised and carried out by specialist palliative care teams. The boundary between B and C is fluid. Recognising this, recent initiatives of the Australian Government's National Palliative Care Program, including but not limited to the Australian Palliative Residential Aged Care Project (APRAC) and PEPA referred to above, have aimed at increasing the capacity of primary caregivers to work across this boundary, offering care informed by a palliative approach. In coming years we can expect that specialist palliative care services will increase consultancy and limit

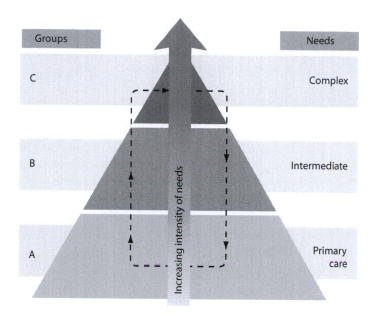

Figure 4.1 Conceptual model of level of need within the population of patients with a life limiting illness (source: Palliative Care Australia 2005).

direct service provision to complex cases, while a growing number of primary care practitioners will be involved in care using a palliative approach.

The strength of this model is that it widens the scope and influence of palliative care through an approach that in principle makes appropriate care for life-limiting illness more accessible to the whole society. The risk of this strategy, from an Ottawa Charter public health perspective (WHO 1986), is that it may reinforce the idea of palliative care as clinical symptom control if its interest is limited to professional service development and the effective provision of those services. A fundamental problem with the model from a public health perspective is that it is concerned not with Australia's population in general but with a specific sub-section of the population – people living with a diagnosis of life-limiting illness who are potentially candidates for palliative care. It is actually a health services, more than a population health, approach.

A comprehensive population health approach should deal with the whole population. Thus the base of the pyramid in Figure 4.1 should be much broader. Below groups A, B and C, there is a group D comprising the rest of the population who do not as yet have a diagnosis of a life-limiting illness, but who will nevertheless in due course require end of life services, for themselves or for their colleagues, friends and families. These services may not be palliative care services as such, but they may be grouped with palliative care under the broader rubric of end of life services. Nearly all of those currently in group D will in due course enter groups A, B or C – but the resources with which they enter palliative care or any other end of life service will depend upon the public health strategies we put in place now. The effectiveness and sustainability of palliative care will depend upon the capacity of the general community to care for their own and to make informed decisions concerning end of life services.

The Australian health care system

A further factor that shapes the reception of policy and program initiative in Australia is the structure of the Australian health system. This is complex, with both public and private funders and providers. The Australian (federal) government has a national role in policy-making but funds, rather than provides, health services. It administers a national insurance scheme, Medicare, that subsidises medical services, and a Pharmaceutical Benefits Scheme that subsidises the cost of essential drugs. It also provides funds to state governments, through the Australian Health Care Agreements, to run public hospitals (Healy *et al.* 2006).

The states have significant autonomy in administering health services, subject of course to intergovernmental agreements, and thus policies, administrative structures, and resource distribution can vary from state to state. Palliative care policy, funding and services certainly vary across the states. While funding is provided through the National Palliative Care Program, only part of this is distributed through national programs. The majority is allocated through the Health Care Agreements with the states. Some states, such as Victoria, fund a diverse network of dedicated palliative care services. Other states, such as New South Wales, fund some specialist palliative care services, but allocate a significant proportion of palliative care money to Area Health Services that then distribute this through a variety of relevant networks. The management structures of palliative care also differ between states. In Western Australia palliative care is linked into a Cancer and Palliative Care Network. In Victoria until recently palliative care was located within aged care, despite the fact that the majority of palliative care at the time was directed toward cancer: as palliative care began to attend to aged care and illness beyond cancer, the palliative care section was relocated with Integrated Cancer Services. Now cancer and palliative care are part of the Division of Well-Being, Integrated Care and Ageing. Federally, the palliative care section was until recently part of the Rural Health Division. Palliative care is not the only area subject to these variations: public health shows analogous variations across state and federal structures (Lin *et al.* 2007, p. 50–57). It is not surprising, then, that most policy implementation begins with projects undertaken within state boundaries; and that care must be taken in translating the details of any particular program across state boundaries. It also follows that policy conversations between palliative care and public health organisations at a national level may take a somewhat different form when continued at state level.

Ways ahead: community capacity building

Community capacity building is a term being used at both state and federal levels in an attempt to bring together public health and needs-based population health approaches. Elements of a community capacity building approach already present within Australian palliative care include:

- A tradition of community activism in creating hospice care networks, continued to an extent in the involvement of community volunteers in palliative care.
- Social marketing carried out by Palliative Care Australia and state palliative care bodies to raise the awareness of palliative care services among the general population.
- National training programs that train primary care practitioners in the philosophy and skills of palliative care, providing a basis for innovative palliative approaches in a range of community settings.
- An awareness among palliative care associations and a number of specialist services of the need for community development approaches; and some projects that express this.

To build upon this foundation we need partnerships that bridge between specialist palliative care services, primary care networks, and community organisations. To date we have focused more upon offering palliative care knowledge and skills to interested individual primary care practitioners than upon forming strategic alliances or partnerships with the commonwealth, state and local government policy frameworks and programs within which these practitioners work. The relationships initiated through palliative approach programs and PEPA are an excellent starting point: but they need to lead on to strategic and policy partnerships. Similarly, while public health approaches have found a place in policy directed toward specialist palliative care services, the next step in implementation is to develop the public health dimensions of a palliative approach, which will include, among other things, building multi-disciplinary primary care networks to implement whole-person care.

These models – HPPC, the palliative approach, and a needs-based approach – take differing approaches to community capacity building. HPPC has focused on local community development initiatives undertaken by specialist palliative care services. The palliative approach has focused on equipping primary health care practitioners, particularly in residential aged care facilities. The needs-based model identifies palliative care as a component of most primary practitioners' activities. Ideally community capacity building approaches will incorporate public health perspectives and projects into palliative approaches that at the moment focus predominantly on professional practice; and direct the attention of health promoting approaches to partnerships with health providers as well as other community groups.

Approaches to community capacity building

In a review of community development approaches, Kellehear (2005, pp. 117–136) identifies four models commonly used in health care settings. These are summarised in Table 4.1.

All four models have their place in community capacity building. The 'healthy cities' model focuses on change through policy development; the community development approach employs a designated worker to develop and strengthen community networks in support of particular health initiatives; the community-focused professional is already a practitioner in the community who adds a community development role to his or her current practice; while the community activist is a person outside the health system as such who has, for one reason or another, a deep concern about a particular health issue. Obviously there is overlap between the models and synchronicity between the various participants. In Hume Region's Caring Communities Project, for example, a project worker whose role combined that of a community development worker and a community-focused professional coordinated a team of community-focused professionals who, in their turn, supported community activists to realise some of their plans for community events and programs addressing dying and loss (Salau et al. 2007). Clearly also the effectiveness of community development is conditioned by the receptivity of the community organisation (Kenny 1999, p. 283) in which it is undertaken.

There is in fact a wealth of resources for community capacity building available from general health promotion and community development sources: integrated models, management strategies, practice tools, evaluation frameworks are there to be adapted for use in palliative care capacity building. However, doing so effectively requires partnerships between the sectors.

A fundamental issue to be addressed in building partnerships is the conceptual dissonance between health services models and public health approaches to palliative care that has already been noted. The issue is not peculiar to palliative care. Within public health practice, for example, there is a similar dissonance between individualist health promotion and structural-collectivist health

Table 4.1 Community development models used in health care

Model	Aim	Role	Skills
Healthy cities	Policy change	Statutory	Corporate
Community development	Extend or transcend services	Employed	Organisational
Community-focused professional	Improve services	Paid activist	Personal
Community activist (unpaid)	Create alternatives to services	Voluntary activist	Political

Source: Adapted from Kellehear 2005.

promotion (Richmond and Germov 2005). The former approach is expressed through programs aiming to persuade individuals to change their lifestyles to reduce their risk of premature illness and death. The latter approach encompasses a much wider range of interventions, including participatory community programmes, legislation and bureaucratic intervention. The former attends principally to individual determinants of health, the latter to social determinants of health. Both are needed: but an individual determinants approach is more consistent with a health services model, and much public health language can be assimilated to it. In contrast, a social determinants approach raises significant structural issues that range well beyond the boundaries of the health system.

Needs-based health services approaches and HPPC approaches reflect the same dissonance that is found within the public health sector. The health services model maintains a clear distinction between state-funded professional interventions and informal care or self-care at community level. New public health models, like HPPC, seek to blur this public–private boundary and develop partnerships between community groups and health service agencies. Health services in general struggle with this. Currently they approach community participation through volunteer programs that invite selected community members, through training and accreditation, to support the practice of professional carers. There is little or no room for community initiative – genuine partnership – in such arrangements. Volunteers are regulated because they are seen as exposing the health agency to risk: they are valued more for their capacity to extend the professional activities of the agency than for any innate or distinctive contribution they themselves may bring. Fundamentally, the Australian health system, with its clear divisions between professionals and laity, institution and community, lacks adequate mechanisms to recognise and enter into partnerships with informal carers. And yet the very health services models endorsed by policy make a solution to this dilemma imperative. In Victoria, for example, a client's average length of stay in a community-based palliative care program is 119 days (Kearney 2008). During that period the client will receive a number of visits and telephone calls, but even in a best case scenario these will not add up to more than 48 hours of contact with professional carers. Thus for 117 days the client's care will be in the hands of him- or herself, family members, friends, colleagues, or neighbours. It is not difficult to see where resources need to be invested to improve the care of people living and dying in the community. One response to this largely-unrecognised need is the increasing number of localised hospice services, funded philanthropically or substantially reliant upon volunteers, that are emerging. Many of these are very much like the original grassroots hospice services, both in their organisational structure and their motivations. They are dissatisfied with state-provided palliative care services, and wish to provide an alternative. HOME Hospice (Chapter 10) is a particular example. And in the same way that the health services of the 1970s and early 1980s would not, or could not, respond to the original hospice networks, so today's mainstream palliative care services struggle to respond to the new neighbourhood or district networks.

Perhaps one way to resolve some of the tensions about the process by which community development should take place, and the way community partnerships should be formed, would be to reach broad agreement on the sort of community we might hope to develop. Kellehear (2005) has described this in some detail. While he outlines an expansive social vision it is likely that local government areas, for example, will want to identify some more modest or immediate goals. These might include communities that:

- Provide informational and educational resources on death, dying and loss.
- Promote health for those living with life-limiting illness and loss.
- Provide training for volunteer caregivers – family, friends, neighbors – concerned with life-limiting illness and loss.
- Fund services that support the social identities of people living with life-limiting illness and loss (tape libraries, IT support, reminiscence groups, biography services...)
- Draw upon the expertise of palliative care and bereavement services to communicate realistic and practical knowledge about dying and loss.
- Ensure that local policy and practice does not discriminate against, but seeks actively to incorporate, those living with life-limiting illness and loss.
- Celebrate the contributions of their citizens before these are outlined publicly, perhaps for the first time, in their funeral services.

Policy

From the preceding discussion three key tasks emerge. Palliative care community capacity building requires:

- a policy framework that recognises and supports palliative care community capacity building and responds to initiatives that emerge;
- partnerships among health care providers and community organisations to extend palliative care practice; and
- local community action to raise awareness and develop community capacity in end of life care; and through partnerships make palliative care practice responsive to community desires and needs.

In Australia we are only starting to build the policy frameworks we need: but we are making a start. To date, policy building for palliative care has been carried out principally by national and state peak bodies (Palliative Care Australia, Palliative Care Queensland, Palliative Care South Australia, and so forth). The federal government and state governments refer consistently to the policies of Palliative Care Australia as guiding principles. State governments however draw upon this policy development work in different ways. West Australia for example has a robust policy built upon a needs-based population model (Department of Health WA 2008), but this has little overt reference to health promotion or community development. Victoria on the other hand, in its

Strengthening Palliative Care Policy 2004–2009 (Department of Human Services 2004), has as its last of seven principles:

Principle 7: People with a life-threatening illness and their carers and families are supported by their communities.

Expected outcomes
- Communities are able to actively support friends, family, neighbors, work and social contacts who have life-threatening illness and their carers and families.
- Community awareness of the needs of and supports for people with life-threatening illness and their carers and families is enhanced through community promotion and education

(DHS 2004, p. 7)

This policy is currently being revised, and it is expected that Principle 7 will not only be retained but will have a clearer and more specific action focus.

National policy statements are thus being used to support a variety of emphases and preferred terminologies at state level. It is important that the community capacity building policies currently envisaged by Palliative Care Australia not only manage the conceptual dissonance referred to above, but also translate consistently in state policy. It is also important that community capacity building policy is developed in partnership with public health and community development bodies. Otherwise there is a possibility that palliative care policy will be shaped in language unfamiliar to the wider public health sector. This could become yet another hurdle to be overcome in building inter-sectoral partnerships.

From palliative care to end of life care

Palliative care is not the only provider of end of life care, or the only body with an interest in end of life policy. Thus while palliative care peak bodies can develop material that will be a basis for government palliative care policy, they can only advocate for end of life policy. Palliative Care Australia, the national peak body, is currently undertaking several initiatives in this regard (PCA 2009). Forming appropriate end of life policy will require wide-ranging discussions within and beyond the health system. An obvious conversation partner at the federal level is the National Public Health Partnership. At the state level, palliative care needs to find a place within public health policy and Primary Care Partnerships frameworks. And these conversations will need to range further afield to engage with all interested parties, including the requested death movement.

Evidence-based policy

Finally, there is an urgent need for evidence as a base for policy formation. Some epidemiological work has been undertaken, notably in West Australia (McNamara and Rosenwax 2007), but as yet end of life needs have not been mapped adequately on a national basis. Nor do we have evidence concerning the social determinants of end of life experience and end of life care in Australia.

Evidence that supports the value and effectiveness of health promoting approaches to palliative and community capacity building in palliative care is also needed. Evidence that community groups are willing to engage with palliative care services in exploring end of life issues is readily available, but the outcomes of such engagement – enhanced capacity to discuss end of life needs, enhanced capacity of local communities to care for their own, better informed palliative care patients – are less readily demonstrated, particularly in the short term. The fact that the majority of public health palliative care initiatives have been carried out with local project funding and evaluated within the project's short time span has limited the evidence available. Currently, however, the La Trobe University Palliative Care Unit, in partnership with Palliative Care Victoria, is carrying out a state government funded health promotion program in three of Victoria's eight health regions. This program has generated resources to be used more widely within Victoria, and in other states if desired, and will continue to inform palliative care policy that is currently under revision. It is further hoped that these regional HPPC programs will be sustainable, allowing continuing evaluation and thus developing a more extensive evidence base (Gardner *et al.* 2009).

Continuing development of public health approaches to palliative care

Experience to date has been that interest in public health approaches has been stronger in regional and rural areas than in metropolitan areas, and in community-based rather than hospital-based program. This is not surprising: rural community health services tend to be both flexible and pragmatic, less immured in the complex lines of accountability that characterise metropolitan and hospital services. Nevertheless, country-city and hospital-community distinctions continue to influence the reception and implementation of public health approaches, and need further consideration when developing policy and providing resources.

While it is relatively easy to identify the policy conversations in which palliative care would like to engage, and the partnerships in which it would like to participate, it cannot be assumed that palliative care contributions will be welcomed. Health care policy and health promotion strategy have for a long time ignored end of life issues except as outcomes to be postponed or resisted: the case will need to be made that it is indeed healthy for communities, and society, to incorporate end of life issues in policy, planning and practice.

The forms of engagement suggested by community capacity building also raise questions about the scope and identity of palliative care. While specialist provision of palliative care is clearly delineated, engagement with the range of life-limiting illness and end of life concerns encountered in primary health practice blurs this specialist identity. Engagement with local community issues and aspirations concerning end of life care will extend this process. Similarly, emerging supportive cancer care policies overlap with palliative care interests, and constructive relationships need to be negotiated. A preferred outcome would be involvement of palliative care throughout the cancer journey, as in UK policy. A risk is that the holistic perspective of palliative care will be corralled at the very end of the journey, as illustrated by current psychosocial cancer care guidelines (National Breast Cancer Centre 2003) that identify spiritual and existential issues as end of life palliative concerns, ignoring evidence that spiritual and existential needs are evident throughout the cancer journey, including survivorship (Brady *et al.* 1999; Little *et al.* 2002).

Resistance to public health approaches continues to come mainly from the conceptual dissonance discussed earlier. Practitioners, politicians, health care managers and citizens who see health in terms of clinical priorities and professional service provision fail to take account of the broader social perspective and are unwilling to risk shifting perspective for fear that funds will be diverted from immediate need and urgent symptoms will be left untreated. A projected move away from directed government funding of palliative care, plus consolidation of hospital and community programs in consortia, risks a renewed clinical dominance of the field. Clear policies, effective lobbying and as much evidence as can be marshalled by palliative care practitioners are needed. Affirmative action supporting public health approaches through targeted funding would be ideal – but are unlikely to eventuate.

There are, however, changes taking place in Australian society that should favour public health understanding in the coming years. At a national level, the challenges of climate change and the current economic crisis are leading to a renewed interest in civil society in Australia, and this is fundamental to participatory approaches to health. A less adversarial relationship between federal and state governments opens the possibility of constructive negotiation of revised Health Care Agreements to minimise duplication and 'buck-passing' between federal and state health systems, ushering in a new federalism that has the potential to bring greater clarity to policy and funding arrangements whilst maintaining necessary flexibility at local level. This certainly is the direction advocated by the report of the National Health and Hospitals Reform Commission (NHHRC 2009a, 2009b), although implementation in the current Australian political climate, with a minority federal government, is far from straightforward. Evidence that drives home the necessity of adopting social views of health is becoming available in accessible form through the WHO Commission on Social Determinants of Health (WHO 2008a), reinforced by the WHO Health Report 2008 (WHO 2008b) that emphasises the need for intentional health care reform under consultative leadership. Within the

Australian health system there is an increased emphasis on inter-sectoral collaboration and partnerships, a climate conducive to the sorts of conversations and initiatives outlined above.

The interim report of the NHHRC (2009a) contained a chapter on end of life care that, among other things, endorsed Advance Care Planning (ACP). (The Commission went so far as to suggest that ACP might be a consumer tool for shaping end of life services.) In the two years since the interim report there has been a significant increase in the number of ACP programs operating in hospitals, residential aged care facilities, and the community. In Victoria, in the regions where the HPPC project is being carried out, partnerships between ACP and HPPC workers are emerging. HPPC skills in setting up constructive conversations about end of life issues are providing a context in which ACP can be introduced. ACP may yet provide a practical interface between public health and clinical approaches to end of life care.

Within palliative care itself, health promoting, population health and palliative approach models are linking end of life care with upstream primary care activity.

Palliative care is being seen increasingly as an aspect of end of life care, opening possibilities for constructive conversation leading to national end of life policy. New skill sets are entering the palliative care workforce – a small but increasing proportion of the practitioners entering palliative care have backgrounds in health promotion and community development, and are interested in using this experience in their new field. National promotion of a palliative approach has developed an objective of including basic palliative care training in most health science undergraduate curricula, recognising that at least occasional involvement in palliative care will be included in most health care practitioners' future practice.

Public health continues to be in many respects a minority discourse within Australian palliative care; but it is sufficiently integrated into the field for it to be here to stay. More than that, there is reason for cautious optimism that, given appropriate leadership and advocacy, public health approaches will continue to shape policy and practice for palliative care, and that palliative care will begin to make a contribution to public health in general.

References

Australian Government Department of Health and Ageing (2004) *Guidelines for a Palliative Approach in Residential Aged Care*, Rural Health and Palliative Care Branch, Australian Government Department of Health and Ageing, Canberra.

Bottomley, J. and Tehan, M. (2005) '"They don't know what to say or do": A research report on developing a best practice support model in the workplace for people with a life-threatening illness and employed carers', Palliative Care Victoria, Melbourne.

Brady, M., Peterman, A., Fitchett, G., Mo, M. and Cella, D. (1999) 'A case for including spirituality in quality of life measurement in oncology', *Psychooncology*, Vol. 8, pp. 417–428.

Colen, H. (2004) 'Palliative Care Queensland Community Development Project 2004' *Social Networks: the triennial newsletter of the palliative care and public health network*, No. 2, March 2004, pp. 3–4.

Currow, D., Abernathy, A. and Fazekas, B. (2004) 'Specialist palliative care needs of whole populations: a feasibility study using a novel approach', *Palliative Medicine*, Vol. 18, pp. 239–247.

Department of Health, Western Australia (2008) *Palliative Care Model of Care*, WA Cancer & Palliative Care Network, Department of Health, Western Australia, Perth.

Department of Human Services (2004) *Strengthening Palliative Care: a policy for health and community providers 2004–9*, DHS, Melbourne.

Gardner, F., Rumbold, B. and Salau, S. (2009) *Strengthening Palliative Care in Victoria: Final Report*, La Trobe University Palliative Care Unit, Melbourne. Available at www.pallcarevic.asn.au/media/1255480909684–1962.pdf.

Healy, J. Sharman, E. and Lokuge, B. (2006) 'Australia: health system review', *Health Systems in Transition*, Vol. 8, No. 5, pp. 1–158.

Kearney, J (2008) Presentation to Psychological, Social and Spiritual Care Forum, held by La Trobe University Palliative Care Unit and Palliative Care Victoria, 19 August 2008.

Kellehear, A. (1999a) *Health Promoting Palliative Care*, Oxford University Press, Melbourne.

Kellehear, A. (1999b) 'Health promoting palliative care: developing a model for practice', *Mortality*, Vol. 4, No. 1, pp. 75–82.

Kellehear, A. (2005) *Compassionate Cities: public health and end of life care*, Routledge, London.

Kellehear, A., Bateman, G. and Rumbold, B. (2005) *Practice guidelines for health promoting palliative care*, Palliative Care Unit, La Trobe University, Melbourne.

Kellehear, A. and Young, B. (2007) 'Resilient Communities' in B. Monroe and D. Oliviere (eds) *Resilience in Palliative Care: achievement in adversity*. Oxford University Press, London, pp. 223–238.

Kellehear, A. and O'Connor, D. (2008) 'Health-promoting palliative care: A practice example', *Critical Public Health*, Vol. 18, No. 1, pp. 111–115.

Kenny, S. (1999) *Developing communities for the future: community development in Australia* (2nd ed), Thompson, Melbourne.

Kristjanson, L. Toye, C. and Dawson, S. (2003) 'New dimensions in palliative care: a palliative approach to neurodegenerative diseases and final illness in older people', *Medical Journal of Australia*, Vol. 179, Suppl. 6, pp. S42–44.

Lin, V., Smith, J. and Fawkes, S. (2007) *Public health practice in Australia: the organised effort*, Allen and Unwin, Sydney.

Little, M., Paul, K., Jordens, C. and Sayers, E. (2002) 'Survivorship and discourses of identity', *Psychooncology*, Vol. 11, pp. 170–178.

McNamara, B. and Rosenwax, L. (2007) 'Factors affecting place of death in Western Australia', *Health and Place*, Vol. 13, pp. 356–367.

National Breast Cancer Centre and National Cancer Control Initiative (2003) *Clinical practice guidelines for the psychosocial care of adults with cancer*, National Breast Cancer Centre, Camperdown, NSW.

National Health and Hospitals Reform Commission (2009a) *A Healthier Future for All Australians – Interim Report December 2008*, Commonwealth of Australia, Canberra.

National Health and Hospitals Reform Commission (2009b) *A Healthier Future for All Australians – Final Report May 2009*, Commonwealth of Australia, Canberra.

Palliative Care Australia (2003) *Palliative Care – service provision in Australia: a planning guide (2nd edition)*, Palliative Care Australia, Canberra.

Palliative Care Australia (2005) *A guide to palliative care service development: a population based approach*, Palliative Care Australia, Canberra.

Palliative Care Australia (2009) *EoL – Towards quality care at the end of life*, online newsletter available at www.palliativecare.org.au/Default.aspx?tabid=1951.

Richmond, K. and Germov, J. (2005) 'Health promotion dilemmas' in J. Germov (ed) *Second Opinion: an introduction to health sociology*, (3rd ed). Melbourne, Oxford University Press, pp. 208–228.

Rosenberg, J. (2007) *A study of the integration of health promotion principles and practices in palliative care organisations*, Unpublished doctoral thesis. Queensland University of Technology, Brisbane.

Rosenberg, J. and Yates, P. (2010) 'Health promotion in palliative care: the case for conceptual congruence', *Critical Public Health*, Vol. 20, No. 2, pp. 201–210.

Quinsey, K., Williams, K., Fildes, D., Masso, M., Senior, K., Yeatman, H. and Eagar, K. (2006) *Caring Communities: evaluation of a national palliative care program*, Centre for Health Service Development, University of Wollongong, Wollongong NSW.

Rumbold, B. (1998) 'Implications of mainstreaming hospice into palliative care services' in J. Parker and S. Aranda (eds) *Palliative care: explorations and challenges*, MacLennan & Petty, Sydney, pp. 24–34.

Salau, S., Rumbold, B. and Young, B. (2007) 'From concept to care – enabling community care through a health promoting palliative care approach', *Contemporary Nurse*, Vol. 27, No. 1, pp. 132–140.

Saunders, C. (1996) 'Hospice' *Mortality*, Vol 1, No. 3, pp. 317–322.

Williams, K., Quinsey, K., Fildes D. *et al.* (2006) *Caring Communities: a description of the 37 projects of a national palliative care program*. Centre for Health Service Development, University of Wollongong, Wollongong NSW.

World Health Organization (1980) *Introduction to Healthy Settings*, WHO, Geneva, available at www.who.int/healthy_settings/about/en/

World Health Organization (1986) *The Ottawa Charter for Health Promotion*, WHO, Geneva, available at www.who.int/healthpromotion/conferences/previous/ottawa/en/

World Health Organization (2008a) *Final Report, Commission on Social Determinants of Health*, WHO, Geneva, available at www.who.int/social_determinants/final_report/en/index.html

World Health Organization (2008b) *Now More Than Ever – the World Health Report 2008*, WHO, Geneva, available at www.who.int/whr/2008/en/

5 Public health and palliative care

A perspective from Africa

Julia Downing, Liz Gwyther and Faith Mwangi-Powell

Introduction

Africa is the world's second largest continent, covering an area of 30.2 million square kilometres, and accounts for 14.4 per cent of the global population (Population Reference Bureau 2008). The burden of disease within the region is high: for example, by 2008 there were an estimated 22.5 million people living in sub-Saharan Africa with HIV and AIDS, around 68 per cent of the global burden of the disease (Joint United Nations Programme on HIV/AIDS 2010), and around 700,000 new cancer cases a year (Garcia *et al.* 2007).

This chapter will look at the need for a public health approach to palliative care in Africa, addressing the demographics and scale of the problem and the effect that this has had on the delivery of palliative care services within the region. Examples of implementation of the public health approach from across the region are provided ranging from countries with recent and new palliative care developments, e.g. Namibia, to countries where palliative care is relatively well developed, such as Kenya and Uganda. In addition, examples on issues pertaining to policy, drug access, education and implementation of palliative care within the African context are provided. Such examples draw upon the experiences of different organisations as well as the involvement of various stakeholders including: patients, carers, the community, health professionals, the public and the policy-makers, in the development and provision of palliative care services across the region.

The need for a public health approach to palliative care in Africa

Africa has a higher burden of disease than any other region in the world. There are many interacting reasons for this high burden of disease, which include poverty, low literacy rates, poor nutrition, lack of access to medical care, lack of sanitation. There has also been an increase in non-communicable diseases which can be attributed to a number of factors such as demographic change leading to a rise in the proportion of people older than 60 years, despite the negative effect of HIV/AIDS on life expectancy. Countries in the region with improved income, such as South Africa, experience a quadruple burden of disease comprising pre-transitional diseases (maternal, perinatal and nutritional causes), the emerging chronic diseases, injuries and HIV/AIDS (Bradshaw *et al.* 2003).

A survey on burden of disease conducted in South Africa in 2000 found that the top four causes of death in women were: HIV/AIDS; cardiovascular disease; infectious/parasitic disease other than HIV; and malignant neoplasms. In men, intentional injury was the fourth leading cause of death with malignant neoplasms fifth. The single largest cause of death was HIV/AIDS, accounting for 30 per cent of deaths – five times more than the next single largest cause of death. The burden of these diseases will probably increase as the roll-out of anti-retroviral therapy takes effect and reduces mortality from HIV/AIDS (Mayosi *et al.* 2009).

Table 5.1 shows causes of death in 2002, considering the top five causes of death in five African countries and contrasting against the UK and US.

Access to health care

Access to Western-trained health care professionals is limited because of low numbers of health care professionals, the cost of getting to a health care facility and the cost of health care (Mwangi-Powell *et al.* 2010). People using public health care facilities in many African countries are required to pay a fee at the point of service delivery. This system has been introduced partly in response to pressure from international organisations such as the World Bank and the International Monetary Fund (IMF). Fees at primary health care level are low but may still present a barrier to accessing health care in the climate of extreme poverty that exists in many parts of Africa. Another consequence of fees for service is that many people present late in their illness when the illness may no longer be responsive to cure or may choose not to undertake expensive potentially curative treatments.

The high rates of mortality for diseases where limited prognosis can be predicted and where palliative care would benefit patients and family members are

Table 5.1 Cause of death, percentage of total deaths, 2002 (%)

Cause of death	Country						
	Côte d'Ivoire	*Kenya*	*Namibia*	*Uganda*	*Zambia*	*UK*	*US*
HIV/AIDS	19	35	51	24	42	0.03	1
Infectious/parasitic diseases (exc. HIV)	32	21	12	33	26	1	2
Cardiovascular diseases	11	11	12	8	6	38	38
Malignant neoplasms	4	4	5	3	2	25	23
Intentional injuries	4	2	2	3	0.3	1	2

Source: Adapted from WHO 2004a.

clear from Table 5.1. To date palliative care in Africa has been provided largely by non-governmental organisations (NGOs) responding to community need and accessing finance through grants and donations to be able to offer this service free of charge. However, the large numbers of the population requiring palliative care cannot be reached through informal health care and it has become clear that palliative care must be expanded to reach patients in all clinics and hospitals, including public facilities.

The public health care approach advocated by Stjernsward *et al.* (2007) is a practical solution to expanding the provision of palliative care in Africa. The African Palliative Care Association (APCA) and national hospice and palliative care associations in Africa are working closely with governments to facilitate provision of palliative care through a public health approach. Internationally, palliative care practitioners have developed a framework for palliative care and pain relief to be recognised as a human right (Gwyther *et al.* 2009) and, while hospice and palliative care associations recognise the competing priorities for limited health funds, they also note that palliative care is not a costly service to provide. The key elements for the provision of palliative care are government policies for palliative care, availability of medication for palliative care, education of health care workers, health policy-makers and users (communities) and implementation of services. Palliative care is cost effective care and works alongside curative services – not replacing them (Higginson and Koffman 2005). Indeed, palliative care services in Africa are often the point of initiation of anti-retroviral treatment for patients with HIV. The collaboration of NGOs providing care in the community enhances ease of access to care by taking care to the patients, and the formal health care sector (clinics and hospitals) ensuring access to medication and management of acute problems encountered during the illness facilitates optimal care provision for patients.

The APCA has had particular success in the access to pain medication workshops held in three regions of the continent, bringing together palliative care practitioners, international pain and policy experts, and government health officials to address the issues around access to medication.

The status of palliative care across the region and its impact on implementation

Palliative care in Africa started over 25 years ago with the establishment of the first hospice in Zimbabwe in 1979 (Mwangi-Powell *et al.* 2010). Since then, although there has been marked growth and increased number of providers, access to palliative care is still largely through isolated centres of excellence rather than integrated in the mainstream health care system. Indeed, what constitutes feasible, accessible, and effective palliative care for the majority of those who need the care in Africa, and how to develop such services, remains to be resolved (Harding and Higginson 2005). This statement collaborates a review of hospice and palliative care development across Africa carried out in 2004, which showed that 44.7 per cent of countries (21 out of 47) had no identified hospice and palliative activity and only 8.5 per cent had services approaching integration as outlined by the public health model (Clark *et al.* 2006; see Table 5.2). While the provision of palliative care across Africa has seen marked increase during the past three to four years with new initiatives in countries like Côte d'Ivoire, Angola and the Democratic Republic of Congo, integration into national health systems is still inadequate and provision is still limited in many places to NGOs (Mwangi-Powell *et al.* 2010; APCA 2010a).

To address the challenge of integration and access to palliative care, the World Health Organization (WHO) advocates a public health approach that aims to protect and improve the health and quality of life of the community by translation of new knowledge and skills into evidence-based, cost effective interventions that will be available to all who need them (WHO 1990). This approach is vital for scaling up palliative care across Africa, since statistics show that, for the overwhelming majority of Africans who currently endure HIV/AIDS and other progressive, life-limiting illnesses, access to culturally appropriate holistic palliative care (that includes effective pain management) is at best limited, and at worst non-existent (Harding *et al.* 2007). Consequently the need

Table 5.2 Typology of hospice palliative care service development in Africa

1 No known activity	2 Capacity building	3 Localised provision	4 Approaching integration
	• Presence of sensitised personnel • Expression of interest with key organisations • Links established (international) with service providers • Conference participation • Visit to hospice-palliative care organisations • Education and training (visiting teams) • External training courses undertaken • Preparation of a strategy for service development • Lobbying policy makers/health ministers	*A range of capacity building activities but also:* • Critical mass of activists in one or more locations • Service established – often linked to home care • Local awareness/support • Sources of funding established though may be heavily donor dependent and relatively isolated from one another with little impact on wider health policy • Morphine available • Some training undertaken by the hospice organisation	*A range of capacity building activities but also:* • Critical mass of activists country wide • Range of providers and service types • Broad awareness of palliative care • Measure of integration with mainstream service providers • Impact on policy • Established education centres • Academic links • Research undertaken • National association

Source: Adapted from Clark *et al.* 2007.

for an effective public health approach to palliative care service provision across Africa is a priority. Moreover, given that palliative care is an integral part of care for all patients with life threatening illnesses, it is important that all countries incorporate palliative care into national health systems through the public health approach (Stjernsward *et al.* 2007).

The application and impact of the public health approach to the implementation of palliative care in Africa is varied across countries. This ranges from countries that still have no known palliative care activity such as Gabon, Mali, Western Sahara, and Chad, to mention a few, to countries that have palliative care integrated into national health strategies such as Uganda, Tanzania (under the non-communicable disease policy) and South Africa (APCA 2010a). Other countries, including Rwanda, Ghana, Zambia and Swaziland, with increased advocacy and technical assistance from APCA, are developing national policies for palliative care that will guide future integration into health systems (APCA 2010b). It is expected that such policies will not only ensure that policy-makers, funders, clinicians and community organisations can provide cost effective care that will have significant impacts on the lives of patients living with life threatening illnesses, but will also provide an opportunity for improving the capacity of countries to pull resources and to support the majority of those who need care. A key challenge for the future is to measure the level of policy implementation and how this impacts on patient care outcomes and numbers reached.

Case studies from across the region

Whilst the implementation of the public health approach will vary from country to country, there are key lessons that can be learnt and applied to other countries at similar stages of palliative care development. Case studies of how the public health approach can be implemented in different countries follow, with examples where palliative care has only recently been developed, such as Namibia, to examples of where palliative care is very well developed, such as South Africa.

Namibia

In their review of hospice and palliative care in sub-Saharan Africa, Clark *et al.* (2006, 2007) found that there were no existing palliative care services, although steps were being taken in Namibia to create the organisation workforce and policy capacity for palliative care services to develop. This categorises Namibia as being at the stage of 'Capacity Building' (cf. Table 5.2). At the time there was also no known palliative care training within the country.

In Namibia, there were an estimated 230,000 people living with HIV in 2005, with the adult HIV prevalence being estimated at 19.9 per cent in 2006 (Ministry of Health and Social Services, MoHSS, 2006). It was through the HIV epidemic that home-based care services were set up, many of which had the potential of integrating palliative care, thus enabling delivery and scale-up of palliative care services. In 2006, the MoHSS recognised the need for palliative care in Namibia by employing a Senior Programme Manager for Palliative Care and Opportunistic Infections to take the lead in the development of palliative care. The APCA were also asked to help the MoHSS through funding from the Presidents Emergency Plan for AIDS Relief (PEPFAR). Through this initiative, a programme was developed to scale up palliative care provision through a public health approach that strived to balance quality and coverage (APCA 2008b).

This programme, which is ongoing, aimed to address issues across the public health strategy. A national palliative care task force was developed chaired by the MoHSS. A national situational analysis was undertaken (MoHSS 2010) in order to ascertain the extent to which individuals and organisations are providing palliative care across the country with a view to scaling up palliative care services and the development of comprehensive palliative care guidelines and policies. Palliative care has been included in the National Policy on HIV/AIDS (MoHSS 2007) and work is ongoing to address issues of palliative care guidelines, policy and access to medication.

Members from the palliative care task force attended a workshop on access to essential pain medication held in Namibia in February 2008 (APCA 2008a). At the workshop they drew up a plan for improving access to pain medication for palliative care in Namibia. This work plan included addressing issues around the lack of health care workers trained in palliative care in Namibia; restrictive laws and regulations on who may prescribe, dispense or handle opioids; opiophobia among health professionals and the public; and the lack of availability of morphine at many health facilities. These issues are gradually being tackled, and the task force was involved in the revision of the Namibia Essential Medicines List (NemList) in 2009, in which some palliative care medications have been included.

The lack of trained personnel within Namibia has proved a challenge. Training has been conducted over the past few years, with many nurses and doctors now having received in-service training on palliative care. A programme of integration of palliative care into a home-based care service was developed with Catholic AID Action (CAA), which is now providing palliative care in the majority of its services across Namibia. Nurses, as well as community volunteers, have been trained in palliative care across the country, and several of the nurses are undertaking a Diploma in Palliative Care in Uganda, accredited by Makerere University run through Hospice Africa Uganda. It is hoped that these nurses will develop specialist knowledge on palliative care and be able to continue to take a lead in its development in Namibia. Work has also begun on integrating palliative care into the pre-registration training of nurses and other allied professions. One of the challenges for palliative care training over the past few years has been the lack of clinical placements for trainees within Namibia, thus necessitating the trained nurses to travel to Island Hospice in Zimbabwe in order to gain clinical experience. It is anticipated that clinical placements will in the future be provided by CAA and other organisations as palliative care services develop further in the country.

Advocacy for palliative care within Namibia continues, and the tri-annual conference of the APCA was held in Windhoek in September 2010, thus helping to raise the profile of palliative care within the country. Challenges to scaling up palliative care do exist, but these are surmountable, and there is commitment from the MoHSS to continue to scale up palliative care, addressing issues around policy, drug availability, education and implementation. Whilst palliative care within the country may remain in its infancy, great steps have been taken in its development over the past few years and the development of palliative care in Namibia would now be described as 'localised provision' rather than 'capacity building' (Table 5.2; Clark *et al.* 2006, 2007).

Uganda

In Uganda, over 1.1 million people are now living with HIV, with an estimated 100,000 new infections per year. Of those infected 156,000 require anti-retroviral therapy (ART), yet only about 32,000 are receiving it (Palliative Care Association of Uganda 2009). Both the HIV infection and cancer rates in Uganda threaten individuals irrespective of age, gender and ethnicity. This, along with the need for palliative care, led to the birth of the Palliative Care Association of Uganda (PCAU) along with palliative care organisations and hospital teams. Within the country, the health care system is under-funded and there is typically a wide gap between health care services in the country's rural and urban areas. Therefore, the need to extend coverage for palliative care to all those in need remains a reality.

Access to palliative care in Uganda has increased both in the public and NGO sector since the first clinical services were started in 1993 by Hospice Africa Uganda (HAU) (Merriman 2002). The Ministry of Health (MoH) has played a key role in creating a favourable policy environment for palliative care and, in 2002, Uganda was the first country in Africa to make palliative care a priority in its National Health Plan (Stjernsward 2002; Ramsey 2003) In the *National Strategic Framework for HIV/AIDS activities in Uganda: 2000/1–2005/6*, a section appeared on strengthening palliative care for people living with HIV/AIDS and in support of the recognised need for palliative care within Uganda a palliative care country team was convened in 2002 to spearhead the development of palliative care within Uganda (WHO 2004b).

The MoH recognises PCAU and its partners, such as HAU, Mildmay Uganda, Joy Hospice, Kitovu Home Care, Jinja Hospice, and Mulago Hospital/Makerere University Palliative Care Unit, as important technical experts helping to scale up palliative care nationally. With advancements in the areas of palliative care policy and education and training for service providers, Uganda is one of the countries where best practices in palliative care have been documented by the World Health Organization (WHO 2004b) and many other international palliative care players.

An important part of the development of palliative care in Uganda was that oral morphine was made available in the country from 1993 (Merriman and

Harding 2010). Once available, it was recognised that there are not enough doctors in Uganda to prescribe the morphine: thus it was available, but not accessible. Therefore, the statute was changed that enabled specially trained nurses and clinical officers to prescribe oral morphine, and Uganda became the first country to enable trained palliative care nurses to prescribe oral morphine – an initial evaluation of this programme at HAU showed that nurses were able to effectively prescribe (Logie and Harding 2005), and a more comprehensive evaluation is being planned.

Palliative care is included in the training curricula for health workers, and all doctors who have qualified since 1994 have been educated about palliative care. It is also integrated into many of the nurse training programmes, and specialist training is provided through a diploma/degree in palliative care and a clinical palliative care programme. In 2008 a palliative care unit was developed at Makerere University, providing clinical care at the national referral hospital, Mulago Hospital.

PCAU works within the national framework for palliative care set out in the National Health Sector Strategic plan and is mandated with scaling up palliative care throughout Uganda in conjunction with the MoH. It currently provides technical support and supervision to over ten district palliative care branches/ initiatives to ensure accessibility of palliative care to those in rural areas. Although Uganda has made advances in scaling up of palliative care over the past 15 years, harmonising these efforts, including advocacy, training and education, mentorship, and ensuring standards of care remains a priority. Patients and relatives have also played a big role in spreading news as to how palliative care is helping patients with life threatening illnesses, especially with the control of pain and other distressing symptoms.

In 2008/9, PCAU undertook an audit of palliative care in Uganda to identify and map palliative care provision in Uganda and make recommendations as to where services need to be expanded and scaled up (PCAU 2009). The results showed that, whilst considerable progress has been made in the scaling-up of palliative care in the country and Uganda is seen as 'approaching integration' in terms of palliative care delivery (Clark *et al.* 2007; Table 5.2), only 32 out of the 80 districts (40 per cent) were found to be providing palliative care services, and services were provided by 50 organisations. Some of the ongoing challenges to palliative care delivery included the number of people requiring palliative care, logistical challenges, lack of awareness of palliative care and methods of delivery. Since the audit was undertaken, work has begun to implement palliative care through palliative care teams in the regional referral hospitals throughout the country.

South Africa

The Hospice Palliative Care Association of South Africa (HPCA), hospices and other palliative care providers work actively with the Department of Health in South Africa to optimise provision of palliative care in all communities.

There are a number of different models of care that are used depending on the health care setting.

In the 1990s, South African hospices responded to the needs due to the HIV pandemic and developed the Integrated Community-based Home Care (ICHC) model of care. In this model the microcommunity of the person living with HIV/AIDS, family and friends are supported by the hospice and there is a formal referral system with the other health care providers to ensure that the People Living with HIV/AIDS (PLHA) needs are attended to in a timely manner. The primary carer from the hospice visiting the patient in the home is a community caregiver trained by hospice staff and supervised and supported by a hospice professional nurse. The ICHC programme builds capacity in communities, creates jobs for community members and enhances patient care.

HPCA is using this model as a basis of a new project – Sustainable Palliative Care through Strategic Partnerships. This project invites health care organisations in the health sub-district to form an active partnership to share knowledge and resources to optimise care for the palliative care patient. The project is initiated in each health district through asset mapping of health care resources and resources in social services. The partners identified in the asset mapping formalise an arrangement for inter-referral and training of partners in palliative care.

Palliative care partners have been working with the Department of Health as a steering committee to develop palliative care initiatives within the department. The Department of Health has developed guidelines for palliative care for adults and for children. Alongside this group, an advocacy group has been established by HPCA: the Alliance for Access to Palliative Care. This Alliance is between hospice and palliative care organisations, the Department of Health, academic departments, cancer and HIV groups. The primary aim of the Alliance is to develop a National Strategy for Palliative Care in South Africa.

HPCA has an active strategy of palliative care development and has a goal to develop a palliative care service in every health care sub-district in South Africa. HPCA staff provide structured support and mentorship of NGOs and hospitals to develop palliative care services. A successful hospital based service in the Abundant Life Centre at Victoria Hospital in Cape Town. Hospital staff identify patients who may benefit from palliative care (through the surprise question, 'would you be surprised if this patient died during the next 12 months?' introduced to hospital staff by Professor Keri Thomas of the UK Gold Standards Framework). These patients and family members attend the Abundant Life Centre for clinical psychosocial and spiritual support, and on discharge from the hospital are referred to their local hospice to continue care in the home. Patients continue to visit the Centre as out-patients. This has led to more effective care, appreciated by patients and family members and fewer hospital admissions for patients in this programme.

Through a funding grant from the Canadian International Development Agency (CIDA), HPCA funds 50 hospices throughout South Africa to engage actively with local clinics to provide informal training in palliative care to clinic staff and to strengthen referral between the clinics and the hospice. There are over 400 primary health care clinics in South Africa benefiting from this initiative with the added enhancement in patient care that result from the programme.

Examples of the different aspects of the public health approach

To effectively develop palliative care within a country, it is important that all four aspects of the public health strategy are addressed. Each of these needs to be addressed within the context of the culture, disease demographics, socioeconomics, and the health care system of the country (Stjernsward *et al.* 2007). The following provide examples of countries that have addressed the different components of the public health approach, and from which lessons can be derived.

Policy – Kenya

Since 1984, the Kenyan HIV/AIDS policy environment has evolved through broad phases which, whilst unique to Kenya, reflect the experiences of other countries that had been forced to confront the HIV/AIDS epidemic (Ministry of Health 2003). For example, in 1990 sentinel surveillance data showed that HIV/AIDS prevalence in Kenya was of 6.1 per cent; this information led to significant policy changes in the HIV/AIDS response, with the government declaring that AIDS had become a national crisis (Anon 1993).

Available data also indicate that cancer is increasingly becoming a major cause of death in Kenya. Indeed, statistics shows that in Kenya about 50 people die daily from various forms of cancers and about 80,000 cases of cancer are diagnosed each year (Africa News 2010). Due to multiple factors, including poverty, stigma and ignorance about the nature of the diseases, most patients seek medical aid when the disease is already beyond cure and many patients still have no access to treatment or palliative care (Harding *et al.* 2007). Despite these issues there is no overarching government policy on palliative care, although several palliative care services exist in the country. Moreover, the existing services are poorly integrated into the public health system and oral morphine, the medicine of choice for the treatment of severe chronic pain, is largely unavailable in Kenya's public hospitals (Human Rights Watch 2010).

Indeed, a review of medicines policy by APCA in 2010 showed that Kenya's medicines policy states that oral morphine is an essential medicine that should be a priority for public procurement and available in all national referral, provincial and district hospitals. However, oral morphine is not available in many of Kenya's public hospitals; therefore, this policy has not been realised (APCA 2010b). A wider review of barriers to opioid use also shows that there are regulatory and legal barriers that make access to opioids in Kenya harder and this also includes the taxation of morphine (Harding *et al.* 2007). In addition, there is no government policy on pain management, and no law or guidelines for the medicinal use of opioids (Human Rights Watch 2010). This makes the provision of palliative care through a public health approach a big challenge in Kenya.

With regard to palliative care skills, there is limited integration of palliative care at the institutions of higher learning, and therefore Kenya's medical and nursing schools. Doctors and nurses receive little training on palliative care and pain treatment (Kenya Hospice and Palliative Care Association, KEHPCA, 2010; APCA 2010c). Consequently, health professionals lack skills in assessing and treating pain for patients with life threatening illnesses. At a recent conference with the KEHPCA, the Minister for Public Health and Non-Communicable diseases announced the development of the national cancer control strategy that includes a strong focus on palliative care. This strategy once finalised will provide a good opportunity for fuller integration of palliative care into national health systems in Kenya (KEHPCA 2010).

Drug access – Zambia

The WHO estimates that millions of people around the world are in immediate need of pain management, including those suffering from end-stage HIV/AIDS, terminal cancer, and injuries caused by accidents and violence, as well as surgical patients and children in pain (WHO 2000). Sub-Saharan Africa contributes significantly to these numbers due the burden of HIV/AIDS and increasing cancer cases (Mpanga-Sebuyira et al. 2006). Despite this, however, sub-Saharan Africa has the lowest consumption of opioid analgesics worldwide and while this is due in part to the challenging economic environment and poor health care infrastructure, the failure of many African governments to take reasonable, low cost steps to improve availability of opioid analgesics is a major contributing factor (Human Rights Watch 2010). It is, however, worth noting that a number of African countries have shown progress can be made when governments make an effort to ensure patients have access to pain management services. For example, Uganda has introduced nurse-based prescribing of morphine, which has enhanced access to patients with life threatening illnesses (Merriman and Jagwe 2007).

In Zambia, a considerable number of patients report pain as a major ailment, yet there is limited access to pain medications such as codeine, and even less to morphine. Among health workers and policy-makers, there is an underlying fear of opioids. Moreover, few health care workers are trained in palliative care, and the country has no national policy for palliative care (APCA 2006). Data from the International Narcotics Control Board (INCB) from 2008 show a low consumption of opioids in Zambia and this therefore means that access to medication is still a challenge (INCB 2010). A 2010 policy review by the APCA showed that, although there is no national policy on palliative care and the drug regulatory laws allow for other health professionals to prescribe opioids, most health professionals are unaware of their prescribing rights, thereby impeding access to opioids for medical treatment of patients with life threatening illnesses. Health care professionals are not adequately informed about the legal and regulatory requirements for the use of narcotic drugs and no opportunity has been provided to discuss any mutual concerns (Harding *et al.* 2007; APCA 2010a).

Over the past two years, through advocacy and work of the Palliative Care Association of Zambia (PCAZ), a national strategy to increase morphine availability has been designed and the government has approved the roll-out of morphine across several hospices in Zambia. The programme's key elements are: to increase collaboration among stakeholders; to better train and mentor staff; and to develop opportunities that will increase access to pain treatment and palliative care, while minimising the risk of drug diversion (PCAZ 2009).

Education – South Africa

Palliative care is an integral part of every health care professional's role and as such all health care workers should receive training in palliative care. Unfortunately this is not a reality in most parts of the world. The Alliance for Access to Palliative Care is actively promoting palliative care training for all health care professionals and, through the South African Medical Association, is presenting a course within the Continuing Professional Development programme.

In South Africa, the University of Cape Town (UCT) established postgraduate programmes in 2001 – a postgraduate diploma and a research based Masters of Philosophy in Palliative Medicine. In the early 2000s, UCT was engaged in revising the undergraduate medical curriculum and the palliative medicine teaching staff were able to contribute to curriculum development and to ensure that palliative care was included throughout the undergraduate curriculum.

Graduates of the UCT postgraduate programme in palliative medicine are employed at all South African universities and palliative care is now part of the undergraduate curriculum at all medical schools in the country.

HPCA has been active in advising nursing schools regarding palliative care training and the Deans of the Nursing Colleges have accepted that palliative care is required in basic nursing training. There has been a strong perception that postgraduate palliative care is only required by oncology nurses but HPCA continues to motivate for a stand-alone postgraduate palliative care degree. The UCT Postgraduate Diploma and MPhil Pall Med are now open to all health care professionals, not only doctors.

In 1999, HPCA received a contract from the Department of Health to develop a curriculum for home-based care training. This training would be for non-professional community caregivers and included basic nursing, HIV awareness, counselling skills and palliative care.

A key aspect of accessibility of palliative care is to create awareness of the benefit of palliative care in communities and potential users of palliative care. It is true worldwide that palliative care is a difficult service to promote as people would prefer not to talk about illness, death and dying. HPCA have an active campaign to bring the benefits of hospice and palliative care to the notice of communities and people who may need palliative care in the future. HPCA has partnered with South African sports personalities to promote the service using the phrase 'Have you been touched by Hospice? I have'.

Implementation – Côte d'Ivoire

Côte d'Ivoire has the highest HIV prevalence in West Africa. In 2008, an estimated 3.9 per cent of adults were living with HIV, with regional rates varying from 1.7 per cent in the north-west to 6.1 per cent in Abidjan (UNGASS 2010). The government is strongly committed to an effective national HIV response. However, large gaps remain in the response to the epidemic according to an UNAIDS 2009 evaluation. Risk of infection is still high, especially among young people, and home-based care services for people living with HIV and orphans and other vulnerable children remain insufficient.

Palliative care in Côte d'Ivoire is still in its infancy, with no fully established palliative care programmes. However, there have been a number of government initiatives, in addition to advocacy activities and training for health care workers through a partnership programme between the APCA and Hope World Wide – a local NGO dealing with HIV/AIDS care and management. Launched in April 2007, this partnership is developing a country-specific advocacy program and strengthening networks and links among health and social support organisations to improve the provision of palliative care in this West African nation of 20.6 million people.

Through this partnership, it has been noted that opioids are available in Côte d'Ivoire, including both oral and parenteral morphine, as well as pethidine and fentanyl among the strong opioids. Despite their availability, access is still limited since only doctors are allowed to prescribe opioids, they need a specific prescription form for opioids, and there is complex bureaucracy in obtaining such forms. In addition, the opioids cannot be prescribed for more than seven days (APCA 2007).

With regard to policy, APCA noted that regulation of opioids is undertaken by the government department responsible for regulating all pharmaceuticals and there is no national body or policy that guides the implementation of palliative care or the use of opioids. On education for health care workers, there are limited skills and knowledge of palliative care and therefore there is a huge need to train community and health professional workers, as well as for integration of palliative care into medical undergraduate training curricula.

More importantly, to ensure wider integration of palliative care in the health systems of Côte d'Ivoire, advocacy and sensitisation activities need to be undertaken at the national level.

Conclusion

Whilst palliative care remains relatively new in many parts of Africa, the public health approach to the development of palliative care is integral to ongoing scaling up of services. An approach that aims to protect and improve the health and quality of life of a community by translating the knowledge and skills of palliative care into evidence-based, cost effective interventions available to everyone in the population who needs them is vital (Stjernsward *et al.* 2007).

The exact method of development and service delivery will vary from country to country; however, it is important that we share experiences and learn from each other's successes as well as challenges. In developing palliative care services it is important to integrate palliative care into all levels of care provision from the community level upwards and from the palliative care expert downwards (Stjernsward *et al.* 2007). National and regional palliative care associations have a key part to play in the development and promotion of palliative care within the region, and need to work closely with patients, carers, the community, health professionals, the public and policy-makers in order to develop culturally appropriate, sustainable palliative care services which meet the needs of the individual in their preferred place of care. The public health strategy provides an important framework from which to do this, and despite the challenges faced by many throughout the region, good quality palliative care can be made available to those who need it.

References

Africa News (2010) *Kenya: Cancer kills 50 daily.* www.africanews.com/site/Kenya_Cancer_kills_50_people_daily/list_messages/29886 (accessed 20 November 2010).

Anon. (1993) Kenya: Haggling over Aid for AIDS. *Africa Confidential,* 34 (11).

APCA (2006) *Advocacy Workshop for Palliative Care in Africa, report of workshop held in Entebbe, Uganda, 2006.* Kampala, Uganda. Available at www.apca.co.ug/advocacy/workshop/.htm (accessed 20 November 2010).

APCA (2007) *Advocacy Workshop for Palliative Care in Africa, report of workshop held in Accra, Ghana May 2007.* Kampala, Uganda. Available at www.apca.co.ug/advocacy/workshop/.htm (accessed 20 November 2010).

APCA (2008a) *Advocacy Workshop for Palliative Care in Africa, report of workshop held in Windhoek, Namibia, February 2008.* Kampala, Uganda.

APCA (2008b) *Namibia Project report, April 2008.* Kampala, Uganda.

APCA (2010a) *Annual Report.* Kampala, Uganda.

APCA (2010b) *Review of National Policies across Africa: Project Report.* Kampala, Uganda.

APCA (2010c) *Integration of palliative care in the curriculum of nurses and doctors in four Africa countries: Project Report November.* Kampala, Uganda.

Bradshaw, D., Groenewald, P., Laubscher, R., Nannan, N., Nojilana, B., Norman, R., Pieterse, D., Schneider, M., Bourne, D.E., Timæus, I.M., Dorrington, R. and Johnson, L. (2003) Initial burden of disease estimates for South Africa 2000. *South African Medical Journal.* 93, pp. 682–688.

Clark, D., Wright, M., Hunt, J. and Lynch, T. (2006) *Hospice and Palliative care in Africa: A review of developments and challenges.* Oxford University Press, Oxford.

Clark, D., Wright, M., Hunt, J. and Lynch, T. (2007) Hospice and Palliative care development in Africa: A multi-method review of services and experiences. *Journal of Pain and Symptom Management,* 33 (6) pp. 698–710.

Garcia, M., Jemal, A., Ward, E.M., Center, M.M., Hao, Y., Siegel, R.L. and Thun, M.J. (2007) *Global cancer: Facts and figures 2007.* American Cancer Society, Atlanta.

Gwyther, L., Brennan, F. and Harding, R. (2009) Advancing palliative care as a human right. *Journal of Pain and Symptom Management,* 38, 5, November, pp. 767–774.

Harding, R. and Higginson, IJ. (2005) Palliative care in sub-Saharan Africa. *Lancet,* 365, pp. 1971–1977.

Harding, R., Powell, R.A., Kiyange, F., Downing, J. and Mwangi-Powell, F. (2007) *Pain-relieving drugs in 12 African PEPFAR Countries: mapping current providers, identifying current challenges, and enabling expansion of pain control provision in the management of HIV/AIDS.* APCA, Kampala, Uganda.

Higginson, I.J. and Koffman, J. (2005) Public Health and Palliative Care. *Clinics in Geriatric Medicine,* 21, pp. 45–55.

Human Rights Watch (2010) *Needless Pain: Government Failure to Provide Palliative Care for Children in Kenya.* Human Rights Watch, New York.

International Narcotics Control Board (2010) *Narcotic Drugs: estimated world requirements for 2009. Statistics for 2008.* United Nations, New York.

Joint United Nations Programme on HIV/AIDS (2010) *Global Report: UNAIDS report on the global AIDS epidemic 2010.* UNAIDS, Geneva.

Kenya Hospice and Palliative Care Association (2010), KEHPCA Bi-annual Conference, November 2010.

Logie, D. and Harding, R. (2005) An evaluation of a morphine public health programme for cancer and AIDS pain relief in Sub-Saharan Africa. *BMC Public Health,* 5:82.

Mayosi, B.M., Fisher, A.J., Lalloo, U.G., Sitas, F., Tollman, S.M. and Bradshaw, D. (2009) The burden of non-communicable diseases in South Africa. *Lancet,* 374(9693), pp. 934–947.

Merriman, A. (2002) Uganda: current status of palliative care. *Journal of Pain and Symptom Management,* 24, 252–256.

Merriman, A. and Jagwe, J. (2007) Uganda: delivering analgesia in rural Africa: opioid availability and nurse prescribing. *Journal of Pain and Symptom Management,* 33(5), pp 547–551.

Merriman, A. and Harding, R. (2010) Pain Control in the African Context: the Ugandan introduction of affordable morphine to relieve suffering at the end of life. *Philosophy, Ethics, and Humanities in Medicine,* 5:10.

Ministry of Health (2003) *HIV/AIDS Surveillance in Kenya.* Nairobi, Kenya.

Ministry of Health and Social Services (2006) *Results of the 2006 National Sentinel survey among pregnant women.* Windhoek, Namibia.

Ministry of Health and Social Services (2007) *Republic of Namibia: National Policy on HIV/AIDS.* Windhoek, Namibia.

Ministry of Health and Social Services (2010) *A situational analysis of palliative care service delivery in Namibia.* Windhoek, Namibia.

Mpanga-Sebuyira, L., Gwyther, L. and Merriman, A. (2006) Overview of HIV/AIDS and Palliative Care guide. In Gwyther, L. Merriman, A. Mpanga-Sebuyira, L. and Schietinger, H. (eds) *A clinical guide to supportive and palliative care for HIV/AIDS in sub-Saharan Africa.* APCA, Kampala, Uganda, pp. 1–8.

Mwangi-Powell, F., Ddungu, H., Downing, J., Kiyange, F., Powell, R.A. and Baguma, A. (2010) Palliative Care in Africa. In Ferrell, B. and Coyle, N. (eds) *The Oxford Textbook of Palliative Care Nursing.* Oxford University Press, Oxford, pp. 1319–1329.

Palliative Care Association of Uganda (2009) *Audit report of palliative care services in Uganda.* Kampala, Uganda.

PCAZ (2009) *Roll-out of Morphine in Zambia: Project Report 2009*, Lusaka, Zambia.

Population Reference Bureau (2008) *World Population Data Sheet*. Population Reference Bureau, New York.

Ramsey, S. (2003) Leading the way in African home-based palliative care. *Lancet*, 362 (9398), pp. 1812–1813.

Stjernsward, J. (2002) Uganda: initiating a government public health approach to pain relief and palliative care. *Journal of Pain and Symptom Management*, 24, (2), pp. 257–264.

Stjernsward, J., Foley, K. and Ferries, F. (2007) The public health strategy for palliative care. *Journal of Pain and Symptom Management*, 33, pp. 486–493.

UNGASS (2010) *Rapport National UNGASS 2010 Côte d'Ivoire Janvier 2008–Decembre 2009*. UNGASS.

World Health Organization (1990) *Cancer Pain Relief and Palliative Care*, Technical Report Series 804. WHO, Geneva.

World Health Organization (2000) *Achieving Balance in National Opioid Control Policy: Guidelines for Assessment*. WHO, Geneva.

World Health Organization (2004a) *Cause of death statistics*. WHO, Geneva.

World Health Organization (2004b) *A community health approach to palliative care for HIV/AIDS and Cancer Patients in sub-Saharan Africa*. Geneva, WHO.

6 Public health developments in palliative care in the UK

Steve Conway

> To allow people the deaths they want, end of life care must be radically transformed.
>
> Demos (2010)

Introduction

The above quotation is taken from a recent UK report which emphasizes improving existing end of life care services and creating alternatives to them. It is used here to emphasize an important message: present standards of care in the UK do not meet the social needs of patients and communities. A public health approach, also known as health promoting palliative care, highlights the need for palliative care services to promote and facilitate community engagement and for state intervention within a social model of health. Health promoting palliative care is a growing social movement throughout the world. In the challenging environment of the UK, there are some encouraging developments. This chapter describes the background and rationale for health promoting palliative care, including key demographic, epidemiological and social trends, and it also provides examples of policy and practice developments. Health promoting palliative care draws upon the principles of social justice, equity and 'health for all' from the new public health. Such principles are beginning to be applied in the UK.

The late twentieth century development of hospice and palliative care in the UK and the world wide development of health promoting palliative care have brought some positive developments. For example, fewer people now die in physical pain and the UK recently came first in an international league table for end of life care (Economist Intelligence Unit 2010). At the same time, we also need to recognize that from the turn of the century specialization and professionalization has brought something of an expert takeover of death and dying in ways that have both dehumanized and removed them from everyday experience and consciousness. As this volume indicates, health promoting palliative care offers a way forward. This chapter could not have been written without the help and support received from so many committed people and for this I am very grateful.

Before moving on to discuss the current situation in the UK, it will be useful to describe the main drivers underpinning this. These issues will be discussed as follows:

- quantitative data in terms of recent and predicted demographic and epidemiological trends;
- popular practice around death and dying, especially in response to the collapse in social support caused by social change and an imposed service culture;
- the main tenets of the social movement of health promoting palliative care and its congruence with the progressive history of public health;
- the relevance of a shift towards community engagement and development in public policy generally, including health and social care.

'Hard' quantitative data on demographic and epidemiological trends including the typical age of the dying, causes and place of death is useful to consider in the light of the long-term cost-effectiveness and economic sustainability of current policy and practice.

'Soft' data is helpful in providing facts, which, whilst often staring us in the face, quantitative analysis neglects. Popular practices around death and dying are relevant, especially in response to the so-called collapse in social support caused by social change and a service culture instilled amongst people that is all about other people doing things for us rather than the old fashioned way of doing things for the benefit of ourselves, and for everybody else. This transcends attitude surveys typical of health services research. Whilst such work is very important, geared as it is towards 'customer' or 'client' satisfaction with existing services, exploring social needs around care is neglected in favour of 'needs assessments' or 'health improvement plans' that privilege professional rather than social or community priorities. Services which are not provided or do not meet current targets are therefore simply ignored or neglected.

It is no accident that health promoting care is very congruent with the aims and theories of the World Health Organization's (WHO) Health for All Strategy (e.g. WHO 1978), especially through the philosophy and action strategies outlined in its Ottawa Charter and Healthy Cities programme (WHO 1986, 1996), both of which are elaborated upon in this chapter. A social model of health has a long history in public health; sadly this is neglected in health services research and practice, including end of life care.

Relatedly, it will be useful to outline the main tenets of the social movement of health promoting palliative care and its congruence with new public health approaches that regards social inequality as the root cause of health inequalities.

By way of orientation, it will also be helpful to describe a recent shift towards community engagement and community development in public policy generally, including health and social care. There is no logical reason for considering that end of life care should be exempt from this development. Far from it being an exceptionally sensitive area which is therefore a 'special case', it is a fundamental and universal area of life. Therefore, we can say that community involvement is a special need not a special exemption. As the remainder of the chapter then indicates, changes are afoot.

Each year around 500,000 people die in England and Wales: chronic disease is the main cause of death and over 60 per cent of all deaths are of those aged 65 or above (Department of Health, DoH, 2008). The numbers of deaths throughout England and Wales are expected to rise to 590,000 per year by 2030, including a further increase in the already very large number of deaths in later life and in chronic diseases as the main cause of death (Gomes and Higginson 2008). Most deaths occur in hospitals (around 60 per cent). Furthermore, the experience of acute care services is less than satisfactory. For example, 54 per cent of complaints in acute hospitals between July 2004 and July 2006 related to end of life (EoL) care (Department of Health 2008). Moreover, critical research has described how a distressing or 'shameful' death is the most common experience of dying, not just in the UK but throughout the world (Demos 2010; Kellehear 2005; McNamara and Rosenwax 2007). By 2030 in the UK, and matching global trends, the numbers for those aged 65 and over are likely to have increased rapidly, with 86.7 per cent of all deaths coming from this group, and 43.5 per cent from those in 'deep old age' (85 and over) (Shaw 2006). There are simply not enough direct service resources to cope with this demand and the indications are that resources are likely to continue to shrink rather than expand.

Whilst UK hospices have set a 'gold standard', they only care for a minority: 4 per cent of the dying in England (DoH 2008). The present medical and hospice systems do not have the capacity to guarantee care for the majority of people with life limiting illnesses, or for their carers and survivors. The medical system focuses upon the identification and control of observable and predictable physical symptoms, for example, in cancer services. Other more complex causes of dying are commonly described as 'non-cancer'. In the hospice system an attempt to develop approaches encompassing medical, psycho-social and spiritual care is clearly discernable, with a particular focus upon patients and families.

National demographic and epidemiological trends

The quantitative analysis below provides details of deaths in England and Wales. It was obtained from the Office of National Statistics (ONS) in a series of published tables (www.statistics.gov.uk), the Government Actuary Department (GAD) (Shaw 2006), and from existing secondary analysis of these sources (Gomes and Higginson 2008).

Analysis

Between 1974 and 2003, the total number of deaths from all causes increased for people aged over 64, and for those over 85 it doubled. This reflects a long-term trend that has seen deaths for those aged over 64 as a proportion of all deaths double between 1861 and 2004, with more marked increases for higher age bands within the over 65s. The higher the age band, the bigger the increase as a proportion of all deaths.

From 1974 to 2003, home deaths reduced for those aged over 44 years. The decline was most marked for people aged 75 and over, falling by 13.3 per cent for those aged 75–84 years and 18.7 per cent amongst over 85s. The 'oldest old' (85 and over) died at home less often over the period than other age groups. There has been a marked shift towards more people dying in advanced age (for example, the deaths of over 85s doubled from 16.1 per cent in 1974 to 31.9 per cent in 2003). However, by 2003, only 10.3 per cent of those aged 85 and over died at home.

Between 1974 and 2003, there was an annual average of 138,342 home deaths. The number of people dying in their own home fell from just over 31 per cent in 1974 to 18.1 per cent in 2003. 'Non-cancer' deaths had the most pronounced fall (31.2 per cent and 31 per cent for 'non-cancer' and cancer in 1974 compared to 22.1 per cent and 16.7 per cent respectively in 2003).

There are more female deaths compared to male deaths year on year from 1974 to 2003. For women, deaths at home were always less frequent, and the decline in the proportion of home deaths was most pronounced. The gender gap widened from 3.7 per cent in 1974 to 6.2 per cent in 2003.

Empirical forecasts

GAD calculates that deaths will continue to decrease until 2012, but they will then gradually increase. Deaths are expected to rise to 590,000 annually by 2030. In terms of deaths in later life, by 2030, those aged 65 and over will make up 86.7 per cent and the oldest old (85 and above) 43.5 per cent.

GAD forecasts that if trends in home deaths continue, the number of home deaths will fall steeply and *just less than 1 in 10 people will die at home in 2030*. In overall terms, institutional deaths are forecast to increase by 20.3 per cent. This would mean that by 2030, compared with 2003, there will be 89,473 more people dying in institutions and the bulk of these will be hospitals. Overall, if trends between 1999 and 2003 continue, deaths in NHS hospitals would, in theory, increase by 19 per cent (from 310,815 per year in 2003 to 369,810 per year in 2030; see Table 6.1).

In England and Wales up until the time of writing, more and more people died in institutions (especially hospitals). This is particularly marked for older people and women. This trend appears to be continuing irreversibly within the existing scenario. From 2012, it is projected that deaths will increase substantially. It is predicted that by 2030, the number of deaths in England and Wales will be greater than the number of births (Shaw 2006). In addition, 'non-cancer' patients who have been described as the 'disadvantaged dying' (Poppel et al. 2003) – that is, people dying with non-malignant diseases – presently receive minimal or no palliative care (Ahmed et al. 2004: 536) This trend needs to be considered for future projections. In social terms, the disadvantaged dying can

Table 6.1 Frequency and percentage of deaths by place of occurrence in England and Wales, 1999–2003

Place of death	1999	2000	2001	2002	2003	1999–2003 change
Home	108,086	101,961	98,820	97,485	97,318	−10,768
	19.4%	19.0%	18.6%	18.3%	18.1%	−1.3%
Institutions	448,032	433,703	431,553	436,042	440,936	−7096
	80.6%	81.0%	81.4%	81.7%	81.9%	−1.3%
Psychiatric hospitals	3,809	3,313	3,245	3,043	3,160	−649
	0.7%	0.6%	0.6%	0.6%	0.6%	−0.1%
Hospices[1]	23,104	22,895	22,727	22,891	22,949	−155
	4.2%	4.3%	4.3%	4.3%	4.3%	−0.1%
NHS hospitals	302,076	297,267	297,783	304,405	310,815	−8739
	54.3%	55.5%	56.2%	57.1%	57.8%	−3.5%
Non-NHS hospitals and nursing homes	59,417	55,364	55,825	54,957	54,280	−5137
	10.7%	10.4%	10.5%	10.3%	10.1%	−0.6%
Communal establishments	46,089	41,830	39,676	39,045	38,397	−7692
	8.3%	7.8%	7.5%	7.3%	7.1%	−1.2%
Elsewhere	13,537	13,034	12,297	11,701	11,335	−2,202
	2.4%	2.4%	2.3%	2.2%	2.1%	−0.3%

Source: Gomes and Higginson 2008.

Note

1 Deaths in hospices underestimated by 9.0 per cent. Deaths occurring in 20 NHS free-standing hospices (249 beds of the total of 2779 beds in England and Wales in 2003) do not count as hospice deaths but as NHS hospitals and nursing homes. Therefore, the percentage of hospice deaths in 2003 was likely to be 4.7 per cent and not 4.3 per cent (25,208 deaths instead of 22,249 deaths).

also be considered to include women and marginalized communities. For example, black and ethnic minorities, and older people, are under-represented in palliative care (Ahmed *et al.* 2004: 537–538).

Back to the future: death sociality and community?

In times past, death was a normal part of everyday existence that was managed and took place within the community. However, in many parts of British society, as in many other global contexts, death is becoming increasingly privatized by a politics of individualism and a resulting decline in the availability or use of social supports, e.g. the extended family, the church or the community. The process of rationalization is also a key driver as dying is largely managed through conventional health care services, and there has been a rise in occupational capacity building and expert guidance from doctors, nurses, social workers, psychiatrists, etc. The individualization and secularization of British society, as a reflection of global social change, has meant that institutional and community support for death has gone into reverse (cf. Kellehear 2007). In response, a marked shift towards social support amongst the dying and their carers has been identified in a great deal of social science research (Exley 2004). We might say that death, being the great equalizer, at least in the way it is an unavoidable reality for us all, may therefore throw such imperatives as individualism, rationalization and secularization into chaos and defy attempts to confine it to being an individual affair to be managed by experts and institutions.

Death is the big and unavoidable issue for all of us. It is therefore something of a *general equivalence*. In philosophical terms, death may also be regarded as 'a gift' in that we do not fully understand it or know what, if anything, lies beyond. But these are matters of faith and opinion. Such big questions have been a subject of central concern throughout human history in all cultures and civilizations. However, in factual terms, and as anthropological research shows, death brings an opportunity for regeneration and the continuation of personal and community bonds through individual and cultural remembrance strategies. Whilst traditional death rituals have declined, new forms of them have emerged which reflect social change and the endurance of human social relationships and bonds (Hockey 2011).

It is hard to dispute that throughout history death creates community (Kellehear 2007; Conway 2007). In other words, it has brought people together and communities have managed death and dying themselves. In the past, given the visibility and frequency of dying, it was a normal and everyday part of social life. Death like many other common experiences was a shared event bringing people together, albeit through socio-economic necessity. In past times, death may not have been so well provided for by technology and drugs, but it was much better served by the community. Nevertheless, a growing sociality of death is visible in the present. The social needs of the dying and their loved ones are evidenced in the sociology of death and loss. Such work describes a move towards greater sociality as a means of developing social supports (Exley 2004; Walter 1999).

Health promoting palliative care, social context and social justice

An emphasis upon community, sociality and the use of social resources is of primary importance to health promoting palliative care. From this perspective, health services should work in partnerships with communities of people. This position is based upon the central tenets of a social model of health. In other words, health and illness reveal social characteristics and pre-determinants that, in many ways, are foundational root causes. For example, the large and increasing 'gap' in life spans between the rich and the poor in the UK may be linked with behavioural factors including smoking, 'fatty diets', lack of exercise and so on. However, these causes may also be regarded as symptoms of deeper processes. The underlying factor which typically determines such behaviour is social inequality. Thus, low income, single parenthood, loneliness, social isolation and lack of self esteem reveal key causal processes.

Health promotion in all of the above areas acknowledges the importance of education, information and good local governance, which is participative. The promotion of social justice is longstanding in WHO documentation; for example, it is reflected in the 2008 World Health Report (WHO 2008). As in health promoting palliative care, health and wellbeing are seen as matters of collective responsibility. Kellehear's book *Health Promoting Palliative Care* (1999) integrates the holistic work of Saunders (1987) and others with ideas about health promotion. In particular, community development is a key goal (Kellehear 2005).

The importance of community development

Communities may be regarded as people living in the same area or who share something in common (such as the dying, carers, widows, widowers, etc). Drawing upon the work of Paulo Friere (1972), who is a major influence on community development practice, and the succinct outlines of it by Kellehear (2005) in relation to end of life care, the process of community development can be broken down into these stages:

- consideration of the community's experiences;
- collective examination and identification of the root cause of that experience;
- examination of their implications;
- development of a plan of action.

Community development involves partnerships between professionals and community members and ideally this should be done as equals. The aims of the process are critical consciousness raising, enhancing community resilience and finding creative ways to connect communities with resources

In the UK, community development has typically been drawn upon in initiatives for people living in deprived and marginalized communities (Sure Start,

Health Action Zones, Education Action Zones, New Deal for Communities, etc.). Recent public health initiatives in the UK have used epidemiological data (illness and death statistics) and deprivation index data (unemployment, child protection figures, etc.) to define and target marginalized communities in geographical 'zones'. Indeed, community development has been embraced in governance agendas for tackling health inequalities in the UK (NICE 2008), and throughout Western Europe and in North America (Weiss 1995). In the British context, it is a relatively recent innovation for health services (Jones 1999). Three levels of community development in health services to address social inequalities in health may be identified:

- *Providing direct resources to the community for their development.* This is usually achieved via the work of community health development workers (employing members of the community directly or professional community development workers). The primary goal here is the empowerment of the local community. Other direct resources can include almost anything (cash, services, the creation of green spaces, legislation, etc.).
- *Supporting and sustaining existing community development activities.* This is typically achieved through creating, maintaining and developing an infrastructure to guide and support actions: for example, by providing a safe and supportive environment; via a steering group (including professional and paid community members); by providing clear line management; and through continuous professional development and education.
- *Promoting the community development philosophy* with other colleagues and agencies related to community health. Here the idea is to ensure that the importance and clear understanding of basic community development principles is acknowledged and reflected in the work of others and that it is subject to continuing reflection.

Community development is therefore about supporting and strengthening communities. It strives to broaden and enhance a community's ability to deal with the traumas of death. In short, it seeks to bring about social change and to increase the capacities necessary for its realization. Keeping the principles of health promoting palliative care and community development in mind, the following sections consider examples of public health practice and policy in the UK.

St Theresa's

St Theresa's Hospice in Darlington serves the people of South Durham and North Yorkshire. Public health practice is in a developmental stage.

St Theresa's has worked in local schools on a small scale basis. Following a request from a primary school for help with a bereaved child, a social worker and counsellor visited the school, first meeting the teacher and head teacher. On another visit they lead a question and answer session with the child's class. Here they used prompt cards for children, about 'feelings'. The child was not identified and isolated for special 'therapy'. Feedback was very positive. A similar request came from a secondary school chaplain about a bereaved sixth former. Following several meetings a peer support group was established which aims to provide sustainable social support. Work has also been carried out with a local 'youth inclusion' team. The aim here is to involve as many young people as possible in developing social support strategies around death and loss.

The hospice is also establishing relationships with marginalized community groups. This also includes working in partnership with four local further and higher education colleges to create a Reflections Room as a space for families. This was designed and decorated and furniture was specially made by the colleges, and a local artist provided her services free of charge

Strategic developments

A related and emerging field of public health which could help to reorient palliative care towards the community can be identified at the level of national and regional policy. The recent End of Life Care Strategy (DoH 2008) aims to improve direct services through integrated partnership working, but this also included an emphasis upon 'awareness raising'. Projects which can be linked directly to the strategy include:

Dying Matters

www.dyingmatters.org
This is a coalition of wide ranging public, private and voluntary organizations led by the National Council for Palliative Care that was set up as part of the The End of Life Care Strategy. Its aim is to focus on 'raising awareness' in ways that 'support changing attitudes and behaviours in society towards dying, death and bereavement'. The main focus of the coalition has been health education and information giving. The website is a full of related resources and links to help start conversations in local communities.

Charter for a good death

www.phine.org.uk/group.php?gid=44&page=610
'By a good death we mean one which is free of pain, with family and friends nearby, with dignity and in the place of one's choosing.'
This is the UK's first ever regional public consultation on death and dying. It is linked specifically to the Dying Matters coalition and is part of the public health strategy for the north-east of England. Based upon extensive local consultation, the charter, 'Compassion at the end of life', was produced in collaboration with patients and their carers. The charter is being implemented by the Compassionate Communities Unit at Teesside University which is described in the next section. At a strategic level then, the door appears to be opening for health promoting palliative care.

In Scotland too there are very good signs. The Scottish Assembly have adopted public health and health promotion as priority areas for exploration (National Assembly 2008: 25). This is led by the Scottish Partnership for Palliative Care. A Health Promoting Palliative Care (HPPC) Group – with similarities to the English Dying Matters coalition – has also been set up with representatives from organizations including the University of Edinburgh GP section, the NHS, Scottish Partnership for Palliative Care (SPPC), and several hospices including Chaplaincy representation. The two groups are working together and examples of activities include:

- using media/fundraising opportunities to promote awareness and upcoming activities;
- debate about working in schools with children and parents;
- exploring mechanisms to bring about a 'national conversation' on death and dying;
- a conference on HPPC; and
- working with the SPPC to promote HPPC in Scotland, including suggesting the incorporation of HPPC into its national conference.

Compassionate communities

In the UK, the work described above, developed from the End of Life Care Strategy, is a welcome policy response. As noted at the beginning of this chapter, HPPC has developed as a social movement throughout the world. Most recently in the UK a number of innovative HPPC projects have emerged, otherwise typically described as compassionate communities' projects. This work is based upon Kellehear's (1999, 2005) development of the theory and practice of health promotion outlined in the WHO's Ottawa Charter and Healthy Cities programme, where both strategies are applied to palliative care. The former approach emphasizes the responsibilities of health services as the main advocate of change; the latter emphasizes a broad approach based upon a healthy settings focus which prioritizes partnership across all sectors to empower communities.

Like health promoting palliative care, compassionate communities attempts to bridge the gap between the realities of the widespread 'experience' of distressing deaths and 'practice' which, whilst achieving some notable achievements in standards of physical care, has neglected the social care needs of the dying and their communities or simply ignored it altogether. Compassionate communities is based upon the basic ideas of public health, especially health promotion, and it emphasizes reforms to the way care is conceptualized, organized and delivered. Work that follows a compassionate communities' philosophy is developing in many settings across the UK. This includes the projects described in this book at St Joseph's (Chapter 8) and St Christopher's (Chapter 11) and St Theresa's described above, and other work in Ireland, Scotland and England (for example, Haraldsdottir et al. 2010).

For example, in the Midlands, the Murray Hall Community Trust, which is heavily involved in social care work with marginalized communities and has already produced some outstanding and innovative examples of practice, has formed a compassionate communities' coalition which brings together professionals and communities across all sectors in their area. Indeed, five primary care trusts in the Midlands are funding and developing compassionate communities' projects and evaluations of this work are due to be published in late 2011. A Wellbeing in Dying Group is also connected to work going on in the Midlands and nationally (www.wellbeingindying.org.uk). In Shropshire, Severn Hospice has made links with a community centre and through an NHS funded scheme has developed a compassionate communities initiative. Volunteers from the scheme support those with long-term conditions in their own homes. The informal feedback from both volunteers and those they care for has been very positive (NHS Local 2011).

A further example of such work is the Compassionate Communities Unit at Teesside University under funding from the NHS (www.tees.ac.uk/sections/research/health_socialcare/compassionate.cfm). This is a very recent development but nevertheless worth mentioning as it is firmly tied to the compassionate communities philosophy. This unit focuses on practice, research and policy development. The project is implementing the regional charter for 'A Good Death' in the north-east (mentioned above). The philosophy of this project emphasizes 'the need to normalize death, build public health capacity and aim to create a compassionate community approach to end of life'.

Conclusion

HPPC is increasingly accepted as a valuable framework to support those with life limiting illnesses and their survivors by encouraging, sustaining and resourcing community capacity. The growing incidence of community oriented approaches in a British context should be welcomed and encouraged. Health promotion that focuses upon community development also provides opportunities to increase access to services and address the inequality of the 'disadvantaged dying'. Such approaches also offer alternative resources.

Finally, much work has already taken place on integrating very different perspectives and powers to facilitate effective partnership working between ordinary people, professionals and social scientists/community development workers in palliative care (Kellehear 2005; Conway 2008, 2011). The move towards a social model of palliative care in the UK, whilst by no means a 'finished article', is a step in such a positive direction. There is now a wealth of literature on lay knowledge of health and community, such as in older people's beliefs (Conway 2003, 2004), lay and medical narratives (Kleinman 1988), and cultures (Helman 1986), and health promotion (Catford 1999). Such work serves as useful and practical approaches in different areas of health and medical care. These are useful and important lessons which indicate positive signs for the challenges ahead.

96   S. Conway

References

Ahmed, N., Bestall, J.C., Ahmedzai, S.H., Payne, S.A., Clark, D. and Noble, B. (2004) Systematic review of the problems and issues of accessing specialist palliative care by patients, carers and health and social care professionals. *Palliative Medicine*, 18: 525–542.

Catford, J. (1999) WHO is making a difference through health promotion. *Health Promotion International*, 14(1): 1–4.

Conway, S. (2003) Ageing and imagined community: some cultural constructions and reconstructions. *Sociological Research Online*, 8 Available at www.socresonline.org.uk/8/2/conway.html

Conway, S. (2004 Agency in the context of loss and bereavement: a moral economy of aging? In E. Tulle (ed.) *Old age and agency*, New York: Nova Science Publishers.

Conway, S. (2007) The changing face of death: implications for public health. *Critical Public Health*, 17: 195–202.

Conway, S. (2008) Public health and palliative care: principles into practice? *Critical Public Health*, 18(3): 405–415.

Conway, S. (ed.) (2011) *Governing Death and Loss: Empowerment, involvement and participation*, Oxford: Oxford University Press.

Demos (2010) *Dying for Change*, London: Demos.

Department of Health (2008) *End of Life Care Strategy: Promoting high quality care for all adults at the end of life*, London: HMSO.

Economist Intelligence Unit. (2010) *The quality of death: ranking end-of-life care across the world*. Available at www.eiu.com/sponsor/lienfoundation/qualityofdeath (accessed 4 March 2011).

Exley, C. (2004). Review article: The sociology of dying, death and bereavement. *The Sociology of Health and Illness*, 26: 110–122.

Friere, P. (1972) *Pedagogy of the Oppressed*, Harmondsworth: Penguin.

Gomes, B. and Higginson, I.J. (2008) Where people die (1974–2030): past trends, future projections and implications for care. *Palliative Medicine*, 22: 33–41.

Haraldsdottir, E., Clark, P. and Murray, S.A. (2010) Health-promoting palliative care arrives in Scotland. *European Journal of Palliative Care*, 17(3): 130–132.

Helman, C.G. (1986) '"Feed a Cold, Starve a Fever": folk models of infection in an English suburban community and their relation to medical treatment'. In C. Currer and M. Stacey (eds) *Concepts of Health, Illness and Disease: a comparative perspective*, Leamington Spa: Berg.

Hockey, J. (2011) Contemporary Cultures of Memorialisation: blending social inventiveness and conformity? In Conway, S. (ed.) (2011) *Governing Death and Loss: Empowerment, involvement and participation*, Oxford: Oxford University Press.

Jones, J. (1999) *Private troubles and public issues: a community development approach to health*, Edinburgh: Community Learning Scotland.

Kellehear, A. (1999) *Health Promoting Palliative Care*, Oxford: Oxford University Press.

Kellehear, A. (2005) *Compassionate Cities: Public Health and End of life care*, London: Routledge.

Kellehear, A. (2007) *A social history of dying*, New York: Cambridge University Press.

Kleinman, A. (1988) *The Illness Narratives: suffering, healing and the human condition*, New York: Basic Books.

McNamara, B. and Rosenwax, L. (2007) The mismanagement of dying. *Health Sociology Review*, 16(5): 373–383.

National Assembly (2008) *Living and Dying Well: A National Action Plan for Palliative and End of life Care in Scotland*, Edinburgh: The Scottish Government.

NHS Local (2011) *Community helps people with long term conditions*, London, NHS. Available at http://nhslocal.nhs.uk/story/features/community-helps-people-long-term-conditions (accessed 4 March 2011).

NICE (2008) *Community engagement and community development methods and approaches to health improvement*, London: HMSO.

Poppel, D.M., Cohen, L.M. and Germain, M.J. (2003) The renal palliative care initiative. *Palliative Medicine*, 6: 321–326.

Saunders, C. (1987) What's in a name? *Palliative Medicine*, 1: 57–61.

Shaw, C. (2006) 2004 based national population projections for the UK and constituent countries. *Population Trends*, 123: 9–12.

Walter, T. (1999) *On bereavement: The culture of grief*. Buckingham: Open University Press.

Weiss, C. (1995) Nothing as practical as a good theory: Exploring theory based evaluation for comprehensive community initiatives for children and families. In Connell, J., Kubisch, C., Schorr, L. and Weiss, C. (eds) *New Approaches to Evaluating Community Initiatives: Concepts, Methods and Contexts*, Washington DC: The Aspen Institute.

World Health Organization (1978) *Declaration of Alma-Ata*, Geneva: WHO.

World Health Organization (1986) Ottawa charter for health promotion. *Health Promotion*, 1(4): i–v.

World Health Organization (1996) *Creating Healthy cities in the 21st Century*, Geneva: WHO.

World Health Organization (2008) *The World Health Report 2008: Primary Health Care Now More Than Ever*, Geneva: WHO.

7 Public health approaches to palliative care

The Neighbourhood Network in Kerala

Suresh Kumar

Introduction

There were rapid advances in the field of health in the last century as a result of improved public health measures and the advancement of medical technology. This has generated great hopes for the future. The advances in technology often also create unrealistic expectations about technological power and the benefits of longevity of life. Over the last century, 'medicalisation' and changes in relationships in society have affected traditional ways of dealing with illness and death in communities (Charlton *et al.* 1995). In addition, rapidly increasing costs and the commercialisation of health care services are making proper health care less accessible to many (Hsiao and Liu 1996; Zhang 2004; Trumper and Phillips 1997; Hung *et al.* 2001). The emergence of palliative care in the previous century was a humane reaction towards marginalisation of the terminally ill and the incurable by the existing health care system (Kearney 1992). Such a philosophy and practice of 'total care' to the group of people 'left out' from the mainstream obviously has relevance to the low and middle income country situation, where a large number of patients lack access to basic services that will allow them to live and die with dignity.

One of the major differences between the care of the acutely ill and the chronically ill is the need for regular lifelong supportive care in the latter (Kumar 2006). The medical establishment, with its hospital-centred services, is geared to look after patients with acute illness. Patients with chronic and incurable illnesses need a regular system of support available in the community. Hopefully, the 'acute care' model may in future, under the influence of a widespread palliative care movement, incorporate the concept of total care for the benefit of patients. However, it is also likely that the palliative care initiatives will be influenced by the wider medico-political situation and become just another medical specialty (Kearney 1992). This is likely to happen when palliative care services, whether hospice or hospital based, follow the conventional biomedical model of health care delivery.

Institution based models of palliative care may not be realistic solutions for the problem when we look at the global situation. Fifty six million people die annually, of which 44 million are in low and middle income countries (Murray and Lopez 1996; World Health Organization 2001). Thirty three million of these dying people will benefit from palliative care services (Stjernsward and Clark 2003). There is an additional huge number of incurably ill people who are not yet terminally ill. The total number of people in urgent need of care and support at any point of time will thus be more than 50 million. All of these people would benefit from palliative care. The present palliative care services cater to only a minority group, very often ending up giving a lot to a small number. A recent publication has noted that only 8 per cent of those who require it are able to access palliative care services globally (Economist Intelligence Unit 2010).

The concept of palliative care has always highlighted the role of psychosocial and spiritual factors in the wellbeing of the incurably ill and the dying. Meaningful palliative care requires a combination of socio-economic, cultural and medical solutions. While this rhetoric is in place, the holistic view is lacking in policy and practices either at national or global level. Despite new initiatives in many countries, the technological progress of medicine is medicalising death more and more, and the gap between the 'good' and the actual death has been widening during the last decades (Clark 2002; Smith 2000).

Most palliative care services are either doctor or nurse led. But when we look at the needs and problems of those with long-term and incurable illnesses, they are also of a psychosocial and spiritual nature. Social needs assume importance especially in the developing world. Medical professionals are ill equipped to address such issues. Issues related to incurable and chronic illnesses are psychosocial and spiritual problems with a strong medical/nursing component. The solutions for these problems need to be explored in the community itself.

Thus, the challenge before palliative care workers in the developing world is to evolve a culturally and socio-economically appropriate and acceptable system for long-term and palliative care, accessible to most of those who need it. This can be possible only if the service is part of a community based primary health care system using local manpower and other resources. Social experiments in palliative care in recent years have demonstrated that it is possible to improve the quality of life of incurably and terminally ill people through empowerment of local communities (Kumar 2007). The role of community participation in putting palliative care on its holistic track has also been highlighted by many authors (Stjernsward 2007; Kellehear 2009). Neighbourhood Network in Palliative Care (NNPC), a community owned program in Kerala, India, is a project that evolved out of a series of 'need based' experiments in the community (Rajagopal and Kumar 1999; Ajithakumari *et al.* 1997).

Kerala

Kerala is the southernmost state in India with an area of 39,000 square kilometres and a population of 32 million. It consists of only 1.18 per cent of the country's land area and 3.4 per cent of the population. In spite of its economic backwardness, Kerala has made remarkable achievements in health almost comparable to that of developed countries. The widely accepted health indicators like crude death rate, infant mortality rate and life expectancy evidence this. Kerala's high statistical achievements in health on the background of low per capita income were first brought to international attention through a publication in 1975 by a group of economists (Raj *et al.* 1975). Since then, this paradox of poor development indices with apparently good health status has featured in development and health policy discourses as the 'Kerala model of health'. Kerala achieved health status on a par with that of the US, spending roughly US$10 per capita per year, while the US spends about $3,500 per capita per year on health care. Kerala's high health status in terms of standard health indicators with comparatively low governmental spending in health care services prompted many analysts to suggest that this 'Kerala model' is worth emulating in other developing regions.

Different explanations have been given for this phenomenon. Prominent interpretations place an emphasis on factors such as the unique socio-political environment in the state, a high level of health awareness due to a high literacy level, an extensive and efficient public health care system, a leading role by non-state actors such as Christian missionaries, and higher accessibility to health care due to better infrastructure at the local level (Ekbal 2000). In this context, a US based sociologist highlighted the role of the highly educated, organised and activist populace which make strong demands on the government (Heller 1999).

However, there have been many concerns recently over a changing demographic pattern and high morbidity levels, the two constraining factors inherent in Kerala's model of health. The maintenance of high morbidity levels along with the highly acclaimed low mortality figures has been a characteristic of Kerala for a long time (Panikar and Soman 1984). A comparison of the share of medical and public health services in the total revenue expenditure of Kerala with the average for all-Indian states shows that, in Kerala, health services (including medical and public health services) had a consistently higher percentage share until the end of 1970s. Since then the difference between Kerala and the other states in the percentage share of health services have declined (Sadandan 2001). Over the past couple of decades, the expansion of the private sector, particularly in rural areas, to fill the vacuum created by the government had a definite bearing on the cost of health care. The rapidly increasing health care expenditure in Kerala is detrimentally affecting poor people's access to health care – the escalating costs of private services and reduced public investments could generate inequalities in access for the poor. A recent study on outpatient care utilisation in urban Kerala points to these inequalities in access despite the expansion of private health care (Levesque *et al.* 2006). The evolution and relevance of the evolving rights based palliative care programme with community participation need to be viewed against this background.

Neighbourhood network in palliative care

The first palliative care initiative with community support in Kerala was initiated in 1993 by a non-governmental organisation (NGO), the Pain and Palliative Care Society, in Calicut (Rajagopal and Kumar 1999). The unit had an outpatient clinic and home care services The community's participation was limited to involvement of a few volunteers in nursing and associated chores within the institution and to the donation of money. (Rajagopal and Kumar 1999; Ajithakumari *et al.* 1997). Although some of the resources came from the community, community involvement in the planning and management of the program was minimal. Recognition of the inadequacies of this model both in terms of coverage and other dimensions of total care led to discussions and experiments at the organisational level.

Attempts to develop a community owned service, addressing the defects of the earlier model, resulted in the formal initiation of a project known as the Neighbourhood Network in Palliative Care (NNPC), in the district of Malappuram in 2001, by four organisations – two already working in palliative care and two working in other areas of social work. Active interactions with patients, family and volunteers from the community resulted, over time, in the replacement of a rather hierarchical doctor-led structure in palliative care in Northern Kerala with a decentralised network of community owned initiatives (Shabeer and Kumar 2005).

In this programme, volunteers from the local community are trained to identify problems of the chronically ill in their area and to intervene effectively, with active support from a network of trained professionals. Essentially, NNPC aims to empower local communities to look after the chronically ill and dying patients in the community. It is inspired by the concept of primary health care described by the World Health Organization in the Declaration of Alma-Ata:

> Primary health care is essential health care based on appropriate and acceptable methods and technology made universally accessible to individuals and families in the community through their full participation and at a cost the country and the community can afford, to maintain the spirit of self-reliance.
>
> (World Health Organization 1978)

Under the program, people who can spare at least two hours per week to care for the sick in their area are enrolled in a structured training programme (16 hours of interactive theory sessions plus four clinical days under supervision). On successful completion of this 'entry point' training (which includes an evaluation at the end), the volunteers are encouraged to form groups of 10–15 community volunteers and to identify the problems of the chronically ill people in their area and to organise appropriate interventions. These NNPC groups are supported by trained doctors and nurses. NNPC groups usually work closely with the existing palliative care/primary health care facilities in their area or build palliative care facilities on their own. Volunteers from these groups make regular home visits to follow up on the patients seen by the professional palliative care team.

The community volunteers identify and address a variety of non-medical issues, including financial problems, identify patients in need of care, organise programmes to create awareness in the community, and raise funds for palliative care activities. They also act as the link between the patient in the community and the health care provider in the institution. NNPC does not aim to replace health care professionals with volunteers. Instead, it attempts to supplement the efforts of trained doctors and nurses in psychosocial and spiritual support by trained volunteers in the community. Groups of trained volunteers are tied to palliative care professionals and health care facilities in their communities. The action plans clearly define individuals' and institutions' roles and responsibilities. In between the reporting to the outpatient clinic/inpatient unit by the patient/family, the local volunteers visit the patient at home, supplementing the visits by the nurse-led home care team. Such visits result in better emotional support, better compliance with medical/nursing instructions, earlier reporting of symptoms to the doctor, and social, including financial, support. In places where NNPC is active, patients in need are identified early. Patients or family are not charged for any service.

Within ten years, the initiative has grown into a vast network of 140 community owned palliative care programmes looking after more than 10,000 patients at any one time. It has a workforce of over 12,000 trained community volunteers, 50 palliative care physicians, and 100 palliative care nurses.

All the palliative care units in the network have outpatient services led by palliative care physicians. The doctor–nurse team that manages these outpatient clinics are employed by the local community volunteer groups. The number of outpatient clinic days per week varies from unit to unit. Patients registered at one unit can also attend an outpatient clinic run by another unit.

Most patients are visited at home by community volunteers. In addition, all the units offer regular nurse-led home care services, supplemented by home visits by doctors. Services offered by outpatient clinics and professional home care units include medical consultations, medicines, procedures like tapping of asietic fluids, and wound care. All the units in the network also offer the following services, in addition to the medical and nursing services.

Food: Palliative care units supply regular food for the starving families; usually as a weekly supply of rice and other items collected from individuals and shops in the neighbourhood. 'Rice for the Family' is an important initiative which contributes to the total care of patients in the region, as the cost of prolonged treatment pushes many families into poverty. By the time the patient registers with the palliative care unit they often cannot afford to feed their family.

Educational support to children: Students tend to drop out at the beginning of the academic year because the parents are not able to afford the expense of books and uniforms. Such children from families of poor patients are supported to continue their education. The support is mainly in the form of books, uniforms and umbrellas when the school opens.

Transport: Patients are helped with transport facilities to referral hospitals. In most situations, this is in the form of a vehicle offered free of charge for a follow-up visit/admission to the Medical College hospital or for an admission to the Institute of Palliative Medicine. The trip otherwise could cost the family a month's income.

Rehabilitation: There is a regular attempt to encourage, train and support patients and family members in income-generating activities. The programmes include support and training in making handicrafts – paper bags, envelopes, etc. – and support in rearing chickens, keeping cattle and setting up small shops. Training workshops are organised for patients. The social rehabilitation programme 'Footprints', supported by students from local campuses in Calicut, has attracted a great deal of attention, as it allows those incapacitated by mental or physical illness to develop skills to become financially independent.

Emotional support: Consistent and readily accessible emotional support is a major component of the 'package' offered to patients and families. Community volunteers are trained to interact with patients and family to offer emotional support. All units try to link their patients with local social or religious organisations supporting the marginalised, and with local government to identify benefits from government schemes (Kumar 2009).

The evolving Kerala model in palliative care

The dynamic process of community engagement has caused the palliative care scene in Kerala to evolve further over the years. The most important feature has been the dialogue and interaction between the state and civil society organisations, which has resulted in policy changes and the involvement of government agencies.

Palliative care policy by the Government of Kerala

In 2008, the Government of Kerala declared a palliative care policy highlighting the concept of community based care and giving guidelines for the development of services with community participation for the incurably ill and bed ridden patients (Health and Family Welfare Department 2008). This document was the result of a series of discussions between the government and the various initiatives in palliative care in the state (see Appendices 1 and 4).

The new policy aims to provide palliative care to as many needy as possible in the state. The policy, which presented short-term as well as long-term objectives, envisages the guiding principle of home based, palliative care as part of general health care and adequate orientation of available manpower and existing institutions in the heath care field. The government has made it clear that the governmental machinery will work in harmony with community based organisations (CBOs) and NGOs which have experience in delivery of palliative care. In practical terms, the document aims at mobilising volunteers locally, providing them with training in palliative care and empowering these trained groups to work with the health care system. The government also expects the Local Self Government Institutions (LSGI) to get heavily involved in this activity.

The policy aims to make community based palliative care programmes with home care services available to the majority of the needy in the state with active participation of CBOs, LSGIs and local health care programs and to develop common bodies/platforms in LSGIs to coordinate the palliative care activities of all bodies and programmes.

National Rural Health Mission (Kerala) project in palliative care

The National Rural Health Mission (NRHM) is a national scheme launched in April 2005. One stated goal of this scheme is to increase total government health spending from its previous level of about 1 per cent of gross domestic product (GDP) to a targeted 2–3 per cent of GDP by 2012, the end of the Eleventh Five-Year Plan (Government of India 2005). NRHM was launched in the light of the National Commission on Macroeconomics and Health (NCMH) recommendation for increased government spending in health (Government of India 2003). Most NRHM funds are routed through state health societies, which have been restructured to incorporate a number of earlier programme-specific societies. The Kerala state health society of the NRHM has been named Arogyakeralam (Healthy Kerala).

NRHM has greatly improved the availability of funds in the government health sector but the trend for the centre to fund an increasing share of primary health care expenditures has also drawn criticism on the ground that it might reduce the states' own accountability for these activities (Bermen and Ahuja 2008).

Arogyakeralam has been involved in palliative care activities in Kerala since 2007. In addition to adding palliative care to the agenda of its grassroot level Accredited Social Health Activist (ASHA), the mission collaborated with Institute of Palliative Medicine in piloting district level projects in the three districts where NNPC has been very active.

Encouraged by the results of the pilot project, NRHM (Kerala) initiated a state level project in 2008 aiming to develop community based care services for the bed ridden, elderly, chronically and incurably ill people in the state. This unique initiative is expected to have wide positive implications in the care of these marginalised groups of people in the state and also nationally. In Kerala, the new project has been instrumental in channelling the energy and resources of a large number of major players, both governmental and non-governmental, to the palliative care and public health scene.

The NRHM project represents the main implementation of the Government of Kerala's palliative care policy. The project, with the Institute of Palliative Medicine as the nodal agency, aims to raise awareness and capacity building in the general community, and among health care professionals in government and private sector, local self government officials and grassroot level political leaders. A series of demonstration projects running alongside these awareness and training activities are facilitating the evolution of the social movement in the care of the incurably and terminally ill patients in the state, which is well integrated to the existing health care system.

Local self government institutions

The Eleventh Schedule added to the Constitution of India by the 73rd amendment lists 29 functions that can be devolved by states to rural local bodies (*panchayati raj* institutions – LSGI). States were free to set the speed and design of their approach to decentralisation under the general framework of the Constitutional mandate. Although the Constitutional amendments were enacted at a central level, it is at the state level where authority for expenditure assignment and devolution of functions to panchayats is fundamentally vested. No devolution of functions is expected from the centre to the states.

The enabling legislation in Kerala constituted the lowest tiers of local governments as autonomous agents of development resulting in a decentralised system of governance, with a three-tier system of LSGI called *Panchayaths*. These LSGI are in charge of important areas like health, education and social welfare. The local self-governments belonging to higher tiers do not have any control over the lower tiers.

As part of the legislation that followed the policy document, the Government of Kerala issued government orders encouraging the involvement of LSGIs in palliative care (Government of Kerala 2009a) and facilitating the collaboration of government hospitals including primary health centres in the process (Government of Kerala 2009b). These, along with the sensitisation and training programmes by the NRHM Palliative Care Project, have resulted in more than 200 LSGI taking up palliative care projects. This number is steadily increasing. It is estimated that the majority of the 1,000 or so LSGI will have palliative care projects in their areas within a couple of years.

A systematic attempt at integrating the existing services was initiated in Kerala in 2008. The evolving 'Kerala model' in palliative care is represented diagrammatically in Figure 7.1.

Conclusion

Programs like NNPC depend on the spirit of generalised reciprocity and trust in society, referred to as social capital. Development of such a palliative care movement based on social capital with civil society organisations (CSOs) as facilitators can hopefully address questions of coverage and quality of services. Palliative care with community participation will hopefully also gain acceptance of economic institutions as an expression of social capital. This will mean 'quantifying' the outcomes and their cross sectoral analyses as a future task of the programme.

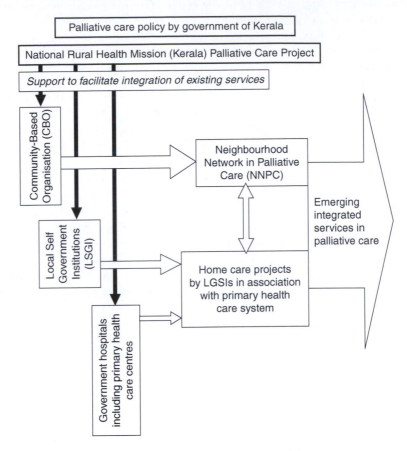

Figure 7.1 Palliative care in Kerala – the emerging model.

The palliative care programme in Kerala has attracted attention for different reasons (Stjernsward 2005), including: the estimated good coverage for palliative care and long-term care in a 'resource poor' setting, the enthusiasm that has been generated in the local community, and the reliance on locally generated funds and hence the potential for sustainability. This particular initiative has also triggered discussions and debates on the 'basic' versus 'specialist' palliative care services (Gupta 2004; Lee 2005; Berry 2005; Graham and Clark 2005).

Community based approaches have recently begun to elicit interest among policy-makers and politicians in a wide range of policy areas (Imrie and Raco 2003; Taylor 2003). Partnership of the state with civil society is now seen by many as a means through which a raft of societal and political ills can be addressed (Hodgson, 2004). The 'community turn' as a strategy and part of the new political economy of the welfare state has also been discussed by authors (Jessop 2002). The NNPC is working closely with the state. Unlike most situations, where the community initiative fits into a slot provided by the state (Imrie and Raco 2003; Taylor 2003), the NNPC has engaged local governments to identify and prioritise local health needs (Shabeer and Kumar 2005). The long-term results of this grassroot level democratisation may be worth exploring.

Understanding of community participation in health programmes will be greatly enhanced if in-depth analyses of specific programmes are undertaken (Cohen and Uphoff 1980). Such studies are important as there is no consensus on the definition of the concept of community participation itself. Community is not monolithic. It is heterogeneous, with wide differences in socio-economic status, educational status, religion and ethnicity (Boyce and Lysack 2000). Since different groups in a community have widely differing needs and priorities, participatory projects can have different impacts in various areas (Nelson and Wright 1995). Community volunteer participation in palliative care assumes surplus time and energy in the community, which may be also be unevenly distributed across society in terms of age, class and gender, and across societies.

The application of market logic to all areas of life can lead to serious deficiencies in services to those with little purchasing power. CSOs may unwittingly encourage this process by facilitating the withdrawal of the state from sectors such as health care and education. The Kerala model of palliative care represents a potential way in which civil society can engage in active dialogue and collaborate with the state to provide comprehensive and sustainable care for vulnerable sections of the society.

References

Ajithakumari, K., Kumar, S. and Rajagopal, M.R. (1997) Palliative Home Care: the Calicut experience. *Palliative Medicine*. 11, pp. 451–454.

Amei, Zhang (2004) *Economic Growth and Human Development in China*. UNDP Occasional Paper 28. Available at http://hdr.undp.org/docs/publications/ocational_papers/oc28a.htm (accessed 20 January 2011).

Bermen, P. and Ahuja, R. (2008) Government Health Spending in India. *Economic & Political Weekly*, 43(24), pp. 209–216.

Berry, P. (2005) Response to 'How basic is palliative care?' *International Journal of Palliative Nursing*, 11, pp. 157–158.

Boyce, W. and Lysack, L. (2000) Community Participation: Uncovering its Meanings In Thomas, M. and Thomas, J. (eds). *Selected Readings in Community Based Rehabilitation Series 1*, Bangalore: CBR, pp. 39–54.

Charlton, R., Dovey, S., Mizushima, Y. and Ford, E. (1995) Attitudes to death and dying in the UK, New Zealand and Japan. *Journal of Palliative Care*, 11 (1), pp. 42–47.

Clark, D. (2002) Between hope and acceptance: the medicalisation of dying, *BMJ*, 324(7342), pp. 905–7.

Cohen, M. and Uphoff, N.T. (1980) Participation's place in rural development: seeking clarity through specificity. *World Development*, 8, pp. 213–35.

Economist Intelligence Unit (2010) *The quality of death: Ranking end-of-life care across the world*. Available at http://graphics.eiu.com/upload/QOD_main_final_edition_Jul12_toprint.pdf (accessed on 30 December 2010).

Ekbal, B. (2000) 'People's Campaign for Decentralized Planning and the Health Sector in Kerala', Issue paper, People's Health Assembly. Available at http://phmovement. org/pdf/pubs/phmpubsekbal.pdf (accessed on 28 December 2010).

Government of India (2003) 'Report of the National Commission on Macroeconomics and Health', Ministry of Health and Family Welfare, Government of India, New Delhi. Available at http://mohfw.nic.in (accessed on 3 January 2011).

Government of India (2005) 'National Rural Health Mission, Mission Document (2005–12)', Ministry of Health and Family Welfare, Government of India, New Delhi. Available at http://mohfw.nic.in/NRHM.htm (accessed on 3 January 2011).

Government of Kerala (2009a) *Local Self Government Department GO No. 66373/D.A 1/2009 dated 02.11.2009.*

Government of Kerala (2009b) *Implementation of Pain and Palliative Care Policy, Circular No. PH 6/068463 dated 29 July 2009*, Directorate of Health Services, Government of Kerala.

Graham, F. and Clark, D. (2005) Addressing the basics of palliative care. *International Journal of Palliative Nursing*, 11, pp. 36–9.

Gupta, H. (2004) How basic is palliative care? *International Journal of Palliative Nursing*, 10, pp. 600–1.

Health and Family Welfare (J) Department (2008) GO(P)No 109/2008/H&FWD Dated Thiruvanathapuram 15.4.2008.

Heller, P. (1999) *The Labor of Development: Workers and the Transformation of Capitalism in Kerala, India.* Ithaca: Cornell University Press.

Hodgson, L. (2004) Manufactured Civil Society – Counting the cost. *Critical Social Policy*, 24, pp. 139–164.

Hsiao, W.C.L. and Liu, Y. (1996) Economic Reform and Health – Lessons from China. *New England Journal of Medicine*, 335, pp. 430–432.

Hung, P.M., Dzung, T.V. and Dahlgren, G. (2001) Vietnam: Efficient, equity-Oriented Financial strategies for Health. In Evans, T., Whitehead, M., Diderichsen, F., Bhuiya, A. and Wirth, M. (eds). *Challenging Inequalities in Health – from Ethics to Action.* Oxford: Oxford University Press.

Imrie, R. and Raco, M. (eds). (2003) *Urban Renaissance? New labour, Community and Urban policy.* Bristol: The Policy Press.

Jessop, B. (2002) *The future of the Capitalist State.* Cambridge: Polity Press: Bristol.

Kearney, M. (1992) Palliative medicine–just another specialty? *Palliative Medicine*, 6, pp. 39–46.

Kellehear, A. (2009) Dementia and dying: The need for a systematic policy approach. *Critical Social Policy*, 29, pp. 146.

Kumar, S. (2006) The chronically and incurably ill: Barriers to care. In *Commonwealth Health Ministers Book*, London: Commonwealth Secretariat Publication, pp. 143–148.

Kumar, S. (2007) Kerala, India: A Regional Community-Based Palliative Care Model. *Journal of Pain and Symptom Management*, 33(5), pp. 623–627.

Kumar, S. (2009) Neighbourhood Network in Palliative Care, Kerala, India, In Scott, R. and Howlett, S. (eds) (2009) *Volunteers in Hospice and Palliative Care*, Oxford: Oxford University Press, pp. 211–219.

Lee, G. (2005) Response to 'How basic is palliative care?' *International Journal of Palliative Nursing*, 11, pp. 156–7.

Levesque, J.F., Slim, H., Narayana, D. and Fournier, P. (2006) Outpatient Care Utilization in Urban Kerala, India. *Health Policy and Planning*, 21(4), pp. 289–301.

Murray, C. and Lopez, A. (1996) *The global burden of disease.* Oxford: Oxford University Press.

Nelson, N. and Wright, S. (1995) *Power and Participatory Development: Theory and Practice*. London: I.T. Publications.

Panikar, P.G.K. and Soman, C.R. (1984) *Health Status of Kerala: The Paradox of Economic Backwardness and Health Development*. Thiruvananthapuram: Centre for Development Studies.

Raj, K.N. *et al.* (1975) *Poverty, Unemployment and Development Policy – A Case Study of Selected Issues with Reference to Kerala*. Centre for Development Studies. New York: UN.

Rajagopal, M.R. and Kumar, S. (1999) A model for Delivery of Palliative Care in India – the Calicut experiment. *Journal of Palliative Care*, 15, pp. 44–49.

Sadandan, R. (2001) Government Health Services in Kerala Who Benefits? *Economic and Political Weekly*, 36(32), pp. 3071–3077.

Shabeer, C. and Kumar, S. (2005) Palliative care in the developing world: a social experiment in India *European Journal of Palliative Care*, 13(2), pp. 76–79.

Smith, R. (2000) A good death. *BMJ*, 320, pp. 129–130.

Stjernsward, J. (2005) Community participation in palliative care. *Indian Journal of Palliative Care*, 11, pp. 111–117.

Stjernsward, J. (2007) Palliative Care: The Public Health Strategy. *Journal of Public Health Policy*, 28, pp. 42–55.

Stjernsward, J. and Clark, D. (2003) Palliative Medicine; a global perspective. In Doyle, D., Hanks, G., Cherney, N. and Calman, K. (eds). *Oxford Textbook of Palliative Medicine, 3rd edition*, Oxford: Oxford Medical Publication, pp. 1199–1224

Taylor, M. (2003) *Public Policy in the Community*. Basingstoke: Palgrave.

Trumper, R. and Phillips, L. (1997) Give me discipline and give me death: neoliberalism and health in Chile. *International Journal of Health Services*, 27(1), pp. 41–55.

World Health Organization (1978) *Declaration of Alma-Ata*. Available at www.euro.who. int/AboutWHO/Policy/200108271 (accessed on 27 Dec 2010).

World Health Organization (2001) *World Health Report*. Annex, table 2. Geneva: World Health Organization.

8 A public health approach to palliative care in East London

Early developments, challenges and plans for the future

Heather Richardson

Introduction

Palliative care is long established in East London, arguably longer so than nearly anywhere else in the UK. St Joseph's Hospice, based in Hackney, has been providing care to people facing progressive and life threatening conditions for over 100 years. The Hospice was introduced by the Sisters of Charity, who came from Dublin in 1905 to provide end of life care for the Irish people dying from a variety of conditions, including tuberculosis, arising as a result of poor living conditions (Winslow and Clark 2005). Over the last century other services have grown up in the area, providing additional help and support to those who are dying or bereaved. These include health teams working in primary and secondary care and other voluntary sector organisations. Their input is augmented by local authorities and other social care agencies. Other players exist too: the police will often support those facing bereavement following unexpected death; teachers in schools work with children and young people who have lost a family member or peer; and community leaders/religious leaders support groups as well as individuals who are traumatised as a consequence of terminal illness or bereavement.

Whilst much progress has been made over the last century to improve palliative care and its accessibility to anyone who needs it, there is evidence that current provision is far from satisfactory in meeting the needs and preferences of those who could benefit from it. This chapter describes a new vision for palliative and related care in the future in East London, its rationale, the work of the hospice and other providers in its achievement to date and challenges faced. Finally the chapter makes some suggestions about how the learning in East London could be of value elsewhere to others interested in engaging in a programme of similar development.

A new vision for end of life care in East London

A public health approach to care, as described in Chapter 1, is concerned with the health of people at a population level – focused on reducing mortality and morbidity, and on improving the health of communities. Pioneers of this approach to end of life care stress its participatory nature of engagement and the involvement of local communities in its planning and implementation. They highlight an amended relationship between care provider and recipient in which health interventions are provided 'with' rather than 'on' individuals and in which professionals are no longer necessarily deemed the experts in deciding what a local community need. In relation to end of life care, Kellehear (1999, 2005) stresses the importance of working with communities in designing their own ways to care for one another, particularly those that are minoritised and by implication little understood. Finally, proponents of this approach confirm the importance of establishing health related policies, rather than those concerned with management of disease.

The vision for end of life care in East London embodies many of these characteristics. Its foundation stone is a population-based approach to plans for related care in the future, acknowledging the diversity of the local population in terms of culture, religion, social and economic make up, and gaps in provision for those who have life limiting conditions other than cancer. In order to meet the needs identified in the local population, it calls for an approach to care in which local people are actively engaged. It seeks their help in planning and providing care, and in identifying opportunities for policy development that will improve the overall health and wellbeing of those living in the area. It brings together community and faith leaders alongside professionals working in the field to identify priorities for care in the future and draws heavily on new partnerships that span health, social care, health promotion, community development, education, law and social order. The focus of these partnerships is to operationalise and make real the goal of a 'good death' for the people of East London. The new vision requires local people to be confident, knowledgeable players within the arena of end of life care and in so doing acknowledges their need for related information and training. It recognises an important role for the hospice as a source of expertise in the speciality but understands equally that there are other players with valuable other experience with whom the hospice will want to work in making the dream of a new approach a reality.

This vision is an emerging one, reflective of growing knowledge and increasingly sophisticated thinking on the part of the hospice and other stakeholders that comes with experience and time. Whilst this can be frustrating for those who seek certainty in terms of an operational policy for a service, it is a recognised and valued characteristic of community development and as such something to be protected. The next section of the chapter describes gaps in current provision that must be plugged and reasons why a new approach to planning and providing end of life care in East London is required.

A case for change

According to Office of National Statistics (ONS) data for 2006, 677,400 people live in the boroughs of Tower Hamlets, Newham, Hackney and the City of London. This population is a rapidly growing one. The Greater London Authority (GLA) estimates that by 2016, the population of these boroughs will have grown by an estimated 19 per cent, rising to growth of 29 per cent in 2026. It is also a very diverse community, and a changing one in cultural, social and economic ways. Data from the 2001 census confirmed that Black, Asian and other minority ethnic (BAME) communities living in the local boroughs of Hackney, Newham and Tower Hamlets accounted for 40.5 per cent, 60.7 per cent and 48.5 per cent respectively of their total populations. Projections of the same data for 2011 increase the proportion to 41.4 per cent, 70.6 per cent and 49.4 per cent respectively (Klodawski 2009).

Local public health reports for these three boroughs indicate that approximately 3000 people die each year of progressive and life threatening conditions, the majority from cardiovascular disease, cancer and lung disease which are responsible, respectively for, 34, 28 and 12 per cent of all deaths (Anderson 2008). An increasing number of these people will live for long periods with their condition, and a proportion of these with more than one condition at any one time. They present with ongoing requirements for care, including those arising as they approach the end of life. Demographic data confirms that this care is unlikely to be provided satisfactorily by family or other informal caregivers for many. Over 38 per cent of households are single occupancy, and even when there is an informal caregiver, there is a relatively high chance that he/she will suffer ill health themselves (ibid.). As a result they will need help from others.

Such care is currently provided by a mix of health and social care staff in the main. There is evidence that, despite best efforts on the part of individual practitioners and a growing commitment by local commissioners of care, this provision is inadequate in meeting patient preferences, inequitable in provision and not always of high quality. For example, nearly over 65 per cent of all deaths in London happen in hospital (National End of Life Care Intelligence Network 2010), despite a preference on the part of most people to die at home (Leadbeater and Garber 2010). Nationally a high proportion of complaints in hospital relate to end of life care (see www.kingsfund.org.uk/topics/endoflife_care/), suggesting inadequacies in care in this context. Stories by local people, particularly those from minority ethnic communities, highlight care for dying people which is often culturally insensitive, supported by research undertaken by professionals working in the area (for example Spruyt 1999). Even where care is deemed to be of high quality by those who receive it, such as that provided by the hospice, this care is only available to a small proportion of those who could benefit from it (Anderson 2008). This inequality in provision on the part of the hospice is particularly marked for those with conditions other than cancer and for some socially excluded or marginalised groups.

More positively, local communities in East London are calling for change, and making suggestions for its improvement. For example, dialogues with local Bengali and Somali people highlight the opportunity to receive information that will help them determine how they would like to die.

After attending these sessions I have spoken to other people in our community about death and dying. I have spoken about the fact that death will come to everyone regardless of whether they are religious or not. Although at first people don't want to talk about it or hear after I explain to them that if we talk about it then we can look at how we prepare, then they understand. Coming to these sessions has helped me to talk about [death] to others. It would be really good to have these discussions on a wider scale, include more people involved in the discussions.

(Khatun and Bayliss 2009 p. 4)

They confirm the value they would place on proactive training to help them to support someone coming to the end of his/her life:

Sometimes we don't even understand what medications someone is taking and why because we can't read. We need support in helping us understand so that we can assist with helping them taking their medication . .

Sometime when a patient needs oxygen, what would we do when it is finished – how do we change it, when do we have to do so? We don't know these things . . .

I think if they educated us in what to expect, and what to do when a patient reaches a particular point during the last stages, what are the symptoms, what to expect and how to deal with it then we wouldn't panic as much. Just educate one member of the family, even the patient then that will help us all deal with the situation.

(Ibid. pp. 9–10)

They also propose a new model of care in which members of the community have a central role in providing care and support to people who are dying, trained and supported by the hospice. For example, someone from the Bengali community in East London suggests:

We need volunteers that can perhaps go with the home care team into people's homes. These volunteers don't have to talk about the illness just provide support to patients and families in their own language because sometimes its difficult for patients or families to talk to either other family members or service providers about certain issues but it's easier to talk to someone from the same cultural and religious background who speaks the same language. That would have really helped when my father-in-law was dying at home.

(Ibid. p. 11)

They make a request for changes in national policy and practice around elements of end of life care, notably the use and nature of post mortem. For individuals with an Islamic faith this is undesirable in most situations (Social Action for Health 2007)

As a result, the hospice in partnership with others has started to establish a new approach to end of life care, reflective of the public health approach. Progress to date is described next.

Progress to date

Engaging local people in discussion about dying, death and bereavement

The hospice started this work by engaging with local people to learn more about their experiences of end of life, their preferences in this regard and how services could develop to improve satisfaction with care for those who are dying and bereaved. Over the past four years, the hospice has worked with a number of communities in East London, including the Bengali, Somali, Caribbean, Turkish and Kurdish and some West and Central African communities. Most recently it has started work with the Orthodox Jewish Community in North Hackney. Drawing on stories, it has gained knowledge about the characteristics of a 'good death' for members of these communities, reflective of their history, ethnicity and religious beliefs. It has learnt about how care should be amended to reflect preferences in this regard, informed local people about the rationale for some aspects of clinical practice and negotiated change to others. Our learning is that people are interested to talk about these difficult issues, despite initial reticence, and have very clear ideas about how they would like to approach the end of their lives. They draw on the experience of watching others who die well or otherwise to inform their ideas and engage in iterative discussion to refine their views. Where open invitations have been extended to local people to come and talk about their experiences and preferences, such as that provided by the People's Platform in East London (see www.healthfornel.nhs.uk/engagement/peoplesplatform for more information about this organisation), the uptake by and interest from the general public has been high. Our conclusion is that many people want to explore these issues given the right opportunity, as a basis for taking more control in relation to their own death or those that they love and care for in the future. It has given us confidence about taking forward a new model in which local people are actively involved in planning and shaping services, and which is focused on their priorities rather than those of professionals.

Finding new ways to promote a dialogue about death and dying

In the UK, as well as other parts of the world, there is a growing acknowledgement of the value of enabling people to overcome a natural reticence to talk about death, dying and bereavement and explore these important issues in advance of their own death (for example Dying Matters, www.dyingmatters.org). In recent years at St Joseph's we have sought to open up related conversations in a variety of ways.

In 2007 a well known British photographer called Tom Hunter and an organisation called Rosetta Life created a number of images which explored how users of the hospice were living at home at the end of their lives. Photographic portraits were accompanied by the words of the participants describing their experiences and, in so doing, hopefully contributing to the debate about how people are living with terminal illness in the twenty-first century (www.performingourselves.co.uk/about/interior-lives-tom-hunter). The films were shown in a number of public contexts including a museum and a theatre, drawing in a wide variety of people who, in the main, were keen to talk about what they had seen. The images which are hung in the hospice continue to serve as an important talking point for visitors and others interested specifically in these pieces of work. We are keen to replicate this activity in the future using other artists.

In 2010 the hospice opened its doors for the first time as part of 'Open House London'. This is an annual event in London in which hundreds of buildings are open to visitors at no charge. The organisers describe it a 'a truly city-wide celebration of the buildings, places and neighbourhoods where we live, work and play' (www.londonopenhouse.org). Over 120 people visited the hospice that weekend, the majority for the first time. We are encouraged by the response to the event and plan to open the hospice again in future years.

Ensuring access to care for all who could benefit from it

Historically we have relied on general practitioners, community nurses and hospital staff to facilitate access to the hospice for those who could benefit from its care. Referrals from these sources have been relatively constant, particularly for our well established services of inpatient and home based specialist palliative care. However, dialogue with local ethnic communities highlighted some failure in this system for particular groups, particularly those socially excluded or minoritised. For that reason we have begun to explore other ways of ensuring access for all within the local population who have needs we could meet.

Increased use of the media has been one strategy. The hospice has a communications plan in which there is proactive effort to encourage local media to feature stories describing its work. For some communities, newspaper coverage is effective in conveying a positive message about the services we can offer; for others local radio is better. In 2010 the hospice, along with the local children's hospice, took part in a phone-in programme on Ramadam Radio, run from the London Muslim Centre (LMC) in East London, focused on end of life care. During the programme the Chief Imam from the LMC telephoned in to confirm to listeners that he supported the work of these hospices and considered them to have an important role within the communities that he serves. Interest in visits to the hospice has increased significantly following this programme.

Another strategy has been to proactively recruit and train new volunteers – 'bridgebuilders' who work between the hospice and local communities. They are knowledgeable about the work of the hospice and are also skilled in a variety of techniques to promote discussion around life, death and bereavement by members of the general public, listening to narratives and using creative arts to achieve dialogue. They are recruited from within the communities and trained by the hospice and a local community development organisation (Social Action for Health, SAfH), which has devised a creative tool called 'colours of life' to help people explore issues of life, death, dying and bereavement (see www.safh.org.uk for a workbook on colours of life). Ongoing support for these volunteers is provided by the hospice.

Increased numbers of volunteers, doing a whole range of tasks are part of our strategy to establish a public health model of end of life care. During 2010, the number of volunteers working at the hospice has increased by nearly 50 per cent, including 28 new volunteers recruited and trained as bridgebuilders. The ethnic profile of the volunteers is also changed and much more reflective of the make up of the local population as a result of a proactive recruitment plan. At the time of writing, just 50 per cent of all volunteers identify themselves as White British and the Bridgebuilders are, in the main, from BAME communities. Informal feedback regarding the experience and development of both volunteers and participants has been encouraging and the majority of the new volunteers have been retained.

It is hard to assess the impact of this work, given its relatively short time frame. However, changes in the profile of the hospice users are encouraging and would indicate that we are more accessible to the population as a whole than previously. In 2006–2007, only 19 per cent of inpatients were from BAME communities. In the first eight months of 2010, this number had increased to 33 per cent; BAME patients under the care of the community palliative care team were higher still, at 43 per cent of the total.

Establishing new facilities and services to promote self management and wellbeing

St Joseph's Hospice, like many other hospices, had created a physical environment for care that reflected its traditional approach to meeting people's needs. New hospice wards opened in 2005, for example, were designed to facilitate the delivery of high quality medical and nursing care with attention to infection control, health and safety and privacy of patients, their visitors and staff caring for them. These physical facilities are supported by related policies and procedures including those that reinforce the specific, focused nature of care provided by the hospice. In 2006 the hospice acknowledged that whilst this environment was appropriate for people who were very unwell and who needed specialist, institutional care, alternative facilities could be valuable for people with lesser or different needs related to end of life care and bereavement. The following five years have witnessed the development of a variety of new physical spaces in the hospice that are much less clinical in nature and which aim to draw the general public into the hospice, increase access to information and social support, and promote wellbeing and self management on the part of individuals diagnosed with a life limiting condition, their families and carers. One area known as 'Finding Space' was described by a recent journalist visiting the hospice as 'a cross between a swanky loft apartment and a café' (BBC Radio 4 Casenotes programme, 1 February 2011). It is a facility available to local people who wish to find out more about life limiting conditions, end of life care and bereavement. A newly appointed information officer is based in the space, working closely with complementary therapists and others, available to individuals, families and carers to advise them about how to stay well physically, emotionally and spiritually in the face of challenges of terminal illness and bereavement. Groups with specific diagnoses, such as heart failure, stroke and multiple sclerosis, meet regularly in that setting, finding peer support and help to continue living effectively with their condition. Services such as will making workshops, help with advance care planning and skill swapping sessions for carers are offered on a regular basis, open to anyone who feels they could benefit from them. In 2010 a conservative estimate suggests that there have been over 1000 visits to this facility, which we expect to double in the next year.

Creating new partnerships

In establishing a new approach to end of life care, the hospice has actively sought to create new partnerships that will help change the experience of dying and bereavement in East London.

One of the key partnerships to be strengthened was that with local communities. Whilst the hospice had enjoyed good relationships with many local people who had used the service themselves or known someone cared for by the hospice there were many groups with whom the hospice had no working relationship (Anderson 2008). This was addressed, in part, by establishing a working relationship with SAfH, a local charitable organisation engaged in community development. It works with marginalised communities towards health improvement and increased well being. It encourages local ethnic communities to participate actively to achieve a state of wellbeing, to tackle related barriers and find solutions. Its underpinning principles include a commitment to work from the basis of peoples' own priorities and concerns and to encourage self determination around health and wellbeing (see www.safh.org.uk for further details). Previous work by SAfH had already confirmed concerns on the part of local people around the management of death in a culturally sensitive way. The hospice and SAfH worked together over a period of four years to engage with local people and establish a dialogue about end of life, in part to inform service improvements. Its staff, drawn heavily from local communities, have been instrumental, also, in introducing local people to the hospice by hosting events and activities in the hospice and encouraging use of it by individuals, for whom care from the hospice could be of value. The other role of SAfH has been to model for the hospice a new approach to engagement and development of care. This learning has been invaluable as the hospice continues to establish new relationships with local communities following the end of the formal partnership with SAfH.

The hospice has also engaged other organisations who share a vision and working commitment to improve the experience of end of life and bereavement. To date the partners have included the project Down to Earth, run by Quaker Social Action, which is a practical service helping people living on low incomes to have the funeral they want at a price they can afford (see www.quakersocial-action.com/downtoearth for further information). Together we are engaged in recruiting and training volunteers who can provide advice to people planning their own funeral or that of someone else. Working with Down to Earth we plan to bring together a broad group of like minded individuals working in East London who are interested to work collectively and strategically to improve end of life care. Other partners we have engaged to this end include Age Concern Hackney and Tower Hamlets, a variety of faith and local community leaders, the police and representatives of the local education authority.

Finally the hospice has started to engage with new groups of potential beneficiaries. For example, it has enjoyed partnerships with young people in schools and colleges interested to explore the experience of dying through discussion with people receiving care at the hospice. To date we have had two cohorts of young people from a local sixth form college who have established relationships with patients in day hospice; we have also enjoyed a partnership with a local primary school whose children visited the hospice on a number of occasions to learn more about our work. A description of our relationship on the website of the local sixth form college highlights its value:

> The project is a win-win for all involved, the patients really value the opportunity to reminisce and pass on any gained wisdom to the students, the hospice staff enjoy having younger people around and the students get an understanding of what's important to people who are dying; this is particularly pertinent for this group of students who want to pursue a career in medicine and for me the key to being a great doctor is seeing the person rather than the disease
> (Sam Turner, Associate Director of Corporate Development and Public Engagement, National Council for Palliative Care, cited on www.mossbourne.hackney.sch.uk/assets/pages/news/enrichment_news.php)

Contributing to policy development

The Ottawa Charter for health promotion drawn up in Canada in 1986, on which a public health approach to end of life care draws, stresses the importance of developing healthy public policy. Early on in our relationship with SAfH, the Islamic communities with which we were working highlighted concerns about the process of certification of death and complications therein, which would often serve to delay same day funerals, required as part of their faith. They also described distress and anxiety about use of post mortems, which inevitably delayed funerals and denied their belief around the sacredness of the human body (Social Action for Health 2007). They were uncertain about how to convey these views to those responsible for establishing related national policy or how amendments might be proposed to policies and procedures already in place. To this end the hospice has been working with members of local Islamic communities, SAfH and other stakeholders to identify the issues and explore possible solutions. A conference at the London Muslim Centre took place in May 2011 to which religious leaders, coroners or their representatives, policy-makers and interested others were invited to explore how policy and practice could be amended to reflect religious preferences around post mortem. One option is increased use of MRI scans, the logistics and costs of which are currently being explored.

Challenges encountered and anticipated

This shift to a new model of end of life care, whilst exciting, has not been without its challenges or dilemmas.

What is the baby and what is the bathwater?

The first is the question of what should and could be changed, and what must be protected in terms of traditional hospice care. St Joseph's provides a much loved and high quality service that has been well used over the years by particular sections of the local population and in response to specific needs. In amending the model it is important that those aspects of its care are retained and nurtured. This is harder to do in practice than might be thought. Hospice care, it could be argued, is an emerging art. As a consequence it is often difficult to know what is quintessential to its provision and what is superfluous. When hospice staff and others are anxious about a new approach, this is often at the heart of their concern. Further work is required at local and national levels to clarify the value of hospice care and its contributory parts. In the meantime work is underway locally to help existing staff and volunteers understand the concept of a public health model and to explore its working interface with existing care provided by the hospice and others engaged in end of life care.

Introducing and working with new beneficiary groups

The introduction of new beneficiary groups presents other challenges. The hospice is familiar and confident in its care of people with cancer. This new model proactively seeks to extend the services of the hospice to people with other conditions, and also to those with none at present, that is members of the general public who are currently well or seeking help on behalf of others. In response the hospice must find new ways of working with them and integrating this new approach with its more traditional services. Practical problems arise, such as how these users are categorised for purposes of data collection. For example, if they are not patients, then should they be registered on our clinical database? If they become ill whilst on our premises, should our medical staff assess them or is an ambulance called as would be the case for a visitor to the hospice? Over the past three years the proportion of people with a condition other than cancer under the hospice has increased from 9 per cent in 2006 to 20 per cent at the end of 2010. This proportion is likely to increase substantially in the future. Practical and operational consequences need to be considered as a matter of priority. In addition, our model of care may need amendment to reflect alternative disease trajectories and different types of need.

Assessment and management of risk

The public health model of end of life care, which provides an opportunity for much greater participation on the part of local communities, arguably brings with it a new set of risks for the organisation, reflective of the involvement of lay people in the care of vulnerable adults and their children. The level and nature of related risks for St Joseph's are yet to be established, as is the model of related risk management to ensure the safety of all involved. Examination of other services that are engaged in this work, for example the befriending service established by Marie Curie in Somerset (see www.mariecurie.org.uk/en-gb/health care-professionals/innovation/The-Marie-Curie-Helper/more details), would suggest that the risks are minimal with good training, support and supervision of volunteers; similar work in Australia confirms this to be the case there also (Kerri Noonan, The GroundSwell Project, personal communication).

Regardless, the model of volunteer management may benefit from review and development as we shift in our model of care and utilisation of volunteers. Sallnow (2011) describes two ways of managing volunteers in UK hospices in her conceptual model derived from an analysis of the literature – one focused on restraint and control, the other on empowerment. She proposes that the approach to management of volunteers will affect the impact of the volunteers on quality of care, the value to the individual, financial savings and wider societal benefits. If the hospice is to encourage active participation for service design as well as care delivery, then it needs to embrace a model focused on empowerment, which liberates volunteers to shape their contribution in response to the needs that they see. In a context so often focused on management of risk, this will be a challenge.

Funding for this work

The public health approach to end of life care is, arguably, an economically as well as socially sound model for delivering increased levels and quality of care to people facing the end of life. It could reach many more people than current specialist services, drawing on the time and skill of lay, unpaid carers, and could arguably enable more people to be cared for at home than has previously happened. Even so, there is no funding for this work in East London. Commissioners are clear that they only wish to fund specialist palliative care from the hospice – focused on resolving complex or multiple problems. They have little interest in funding information or self management services or public education.

In order to refine and develop the model in response to local needs and preferences, funding is required. This is currently being sought from charitable rather than statutory sources.

Next steps

St Joseph's plans to start recruiting, training and supporting volunteers to provide care at home within the next year. This work will, hopefully, be supported by a new infrastructure of staff employed to develop and implement a public health approach to end of life care. Funding applications are underway to support this major development.

It is important that staff working in the hospice and other palliative care services understand the public health approach and ideally reassess their own offerings in the light of what it can offer in terms of identifying and responding to need. In the forthcoming months, efforts will be made to share the vision for a public health approach with staff and volunteers at the hospice and in other related services so that we can together plan for its development and future integration. How great a challenge this will be is yet to be seen.

Conclusion

St Joseph's Hospice is at the start of a journey to explore the potential contribution of a public health approach to end of life care in East London. Through pragmatic review of the current and future needs of the local population in relation to end of life care, it has come to the conclusion that current services cannot meet the level or nature of demand through current resources. A new strategy is required, and one which acknowledges the diverse and changing nature of the local population, its capabilities and preferences in this regard. It has also listened and responded to the interest of other local organisations interested to work collaboratively and differently in the future.

A public health model appears to be an appropriate one. It augments current provision and bolsters early work on self management and wellbeing. It addresses the requirement by local people for increased involvement in care and reinforces aspects of the history of St Joseph's and other hospices around innovation, local empowerment and community engagement. In the current economic climate where resources for health and related services are increasingly scarce regardless of increasing need, it is important we look at alternative models that can deliver care which is value for money.

There is more work to be done to implement it successfully. We need to learn more about the most effective role and degree of involvement of the hospice in this model – drawing on the views and expertise of local people, other partners and organisations further afield that have done it successfully in other parts of the world. Finally we need to monitor the process and evaluate the effectiveness and viability of such an approach in a setting like East London.

Despite these limitations we hope that this chapter serves as encouragement to other organisations interested to pursue this approach to end of life care. It is illuminating in terms of the interest shown by local communities to engage with professionals in amending current provision and contributing to a new model of care. The model of engagement with them is one that is both replicable and applicable to a variety of different communities. The chapter confirms the value of using creative, alternative approaches to increasing access and acceptability of existing care in order that the population as a whole is better served by hospices and other similar organisations. The role of the media and the arts to achieve this, and also to initiate a new dialogue around dying, death and bereavement may be interesting to organisations seeking new ways of helping the local public address this difficult and sensitive issue. We hope our positive experience encourages them to explore these opportunities. Finally the development of new facilities and relationships that have enriched and broadened our model of care and our perspective on a good death and end of life care are ones that other similar organisations might consider too. This journey has been an interesting and existing one for us, and we hope the chapter encourages others to consider embarking on a similar expedition of discovery.

References

Anderson, W. (2008) *Responding to need: St Joseph's Hospice and the population it serves. A demographic and epidemiological analysis.* London: St Joseph's Hospice.

Kellehear, A. (1999) *Health promoting palliative care.* Melbourne: Oxford University Press.

Kellehear, A. (2005) *Compassionate Cities: Public health and end of life care.* London: Routledge.

Khatun, M. and Bayliss, E. (2009) *Engaging in dialogue. Local Bengali and Somali people from East London and clinicians and managers from St Joseph's Hospice talk together about end of life care for Muslim patients.* London: Social Action for Health.

Klodawski, E. (2009) *GLA 2008 Round Ethnic Group Population Projections.* Data Management and Analysis Group, Greater London Authority.

Leadbeater, C. and Garber, J. (2010) *Dying for Change.* London: Demos.

National End of Life Care Intelligence Network (2010) *Variations in Place of Death in England. Inequalities or appropriate consequences of age, gender and cause of death?* Bristol: South West Public Health Observatory.

Sallnow, E. (2010) 'Conceptualisation of Volunteering in Palliative Care: A Narrative Synthesis of the Literature'. MSc thesis, Kings College, London.

Social Action for Health (2007) *Managing Death in the Muslim Community in Tower Hamlets. Improving after life services.* London: Social Action for Health.

Spruyt, O. (1999) 'Community-based palliative care for Bangladeshi patients in east London: accounts of bereaved carers', *Palliative Medicine*, Vol. 13, pp. 119–129.

Winslow, M. and Clark, D. (2005) *St Joseph's Hospice Hackney. A century of caring in the East End of London.* Lancaster: Observatory Publications.

9 The campaign to build a dementia-friendly community

The 100-Member Committee, Japan

Introduction

In Japan, where the number of people with dementia is estimated to have reached 1.7 million in 2005 (out of a population of 127.7 million), dementia is no longer a "somebody else's business" but a big challenge for the whole nation. A person with dementia was once considered to be "someone who lost the ability to recognize anyone or anything," or "someone who did one strange thing after another," and was the target of social prejudice. There have been, however, more and more cases in which the patients themselves participate in symposiums or other events to talk about their own painful experiences and express their desire to stay involved in society in whatever way they can. Studies have shown that the peripheral symptoms of dementia are greatly affected by the attitudes of the surrounding people. This has contributed to a growing recognition in Japan that the society should not leave the care of people with dementia to only medical staff or welfare service providers. It is now considered crucial that residents have a proper understanding of dementia, and can support people with this condition in the community in which they live. Taking these social circumstances into account, the Ministry of Health, Labour and Welfare, together with organizations concerned with dementia, launched a ten-year nationwide public campaign in 2005. It is called the "Campaign to Understand Dementia and Build Community Networks." The campaign has been promoted by an organization called "100-Member Committee to Create Safe and Comfortable Communities for People with Dementia" (in short, 100-Member Committee), consisting of about 100 organizations and individuals, with Tsutomu Hotta, CEO of Sawayaka Welfare Foundation, serving as its chairman. The committee membership includes: 1) intellectuals who are national opinion leaders; 2) enterprises and organizations deeply rooted in the community life including national trade organizations of banks and convenience stores; and 3) health, medical care and welfare institutions with a national network. In their fields they actively support people with dementia and their families, upholding the campaign programs.

The four major programs of the Campaign to Understand Dementia and Build Community Networks are:

1 Nationwide caravan to train one million dementia supporters

Central to the campaign is the "Nationwide Caravan to Train One Million Dementia Supporters." This program aims to train, in the next five years, one million "dementia supporters," who understand the characteristics of the disability and provide support for afflicted persons and their families.

2 Support for the associations of people with dementia and their families

In recent years, it has become more common for associations of families of dementia patients to provide occasions for people with dementia to interact with one another. The program supports such an effort.

3 Care management fully involving dementia patients and their families

This program aims at designing a care management program for people with dementia that fully incorporates the desires and initiatives of the afflicted persons and their families, within the framework of the Long-term Care Insurance System. For example, by having the people with dementia fill in the assessment sheet, the program aims at making the care more person-centered. This program offers courses and reporting sessions on this approach on a national level.

4 Campaign to build a dementia-friendly community

This campaign solicits examples of innovative projects which have successfully built a community where people with dementia can live a safe and independent life. Every year the presentation of awards is held in conjunction with the 100-Member Committee Conference. This initiative is discussed in more detail in the following section.

Campaign to build a dementia-friendly community

Since 2004 we have conducted an annual Campaign to Build a Dementia-Friendly Community, in the course of which we have received numerous submissions from around the country describing wonderful community initiatives. An important concept in caring for people with dementia is that each patient continues living in the manner that suits him or her best and that we continue living alongside people with dementia. This means an effort not just by individual specialists or individual facilities but by each and every citizen, working together with the health care, welfare, and government sectors, to build communities that will support people with dementia. This is something that directly affects you and me. Building dementia-friendly communities means creating communities where you and I can live in safety and security in the event that we might develop dementia. We hope everyone will take a look at these pioneering programs from our 2006 campaign, and, using them as a point of reference, tell us about comparable activities in your own community, sharing the thinking and know-how involved in those efforts. Let's work together to create communities where people with dementia can meet their full potential, and where we can all live together.

1 Facility-school interaction – spreading understanding among the young

Joyful Kakamigahara, Sun-Life Social Welfare Corporation/Gifu Prefecture

Description of activities

Joyful Kakamigahara is a facility for the elderly that includes a special nursing home, a group home, and a day-care center. Over the past three years, a lively interaction has developed between the seniors at the facility and the neighborhood elementary school (fifth grade). The initial impetus for the program came in September 2004, when seniors from the facility participated in the school's community Interaction Sports Day. The seniors joined in the tug-of-war from their wheelchairs as if it were the most natural thing in the world. The seniors unfortunately lost to the children, but everyone was impressed by the enthusiastic way they expressed the frustration of defeat. The program, implemented throughout the year in consultation with teachers at the elementary school, has three parts.

1. Visits from the elementary school to the facility and get-togethers with residents (five times per year). After children are taught about dementia at school, the whole class prepares some recreational activities and visits the facility.
2. Visits to the school from the facility. Residents receive invitations from the children to participate in sports day, community musicals, and the harvest festival.
3. School open house (presentations by children summarizing their studies). Seniors enrolled at the facility and staff participate, as well as the Parent-Teacher Association (PTA).

Positive outcomes

1 THE CHILDREN

The majority of seniors from the facility are people with dementia. Through this direct experience the children gradually learn how to interact with people with dementia. Through trial and error, they have learned to prepare easy-to-understand activities. They also learn to speak slowly, one point at a time. Children who have graduated and entered middle school have begun returning to the facility just to visit.

2 PTA

As the children gain an understanding of dementia, they spread that understanding to their families. Tours of the facility and study groups on dementia are also offered for PTA parents.

3 FACILITY STAFF

Staff have come to appreciate more fully how important it is for people with dementia, and for the staff themselves, to regularly interact with the community.

4 MEMBERS OF THE COMMUNITY

When seniors and staff members from the facility go to the supermarket, people often greet them, saying "You're from Joyful, aren't you? I saw you at sports day."

Reasons for awarding the prize

- To see a natural relationship developing between children and people with dementia, with the children growing up as sympathizers and life companions for the elderly, raises high hopes for the future.
- Instead of being limited to specific events or occasional interaction, everyday exchange between seniors and elementary school children continues year by year until it takes root as something natural and expected. The children's understanding is transmitted to their parents and the community as a whole and contributes to community networking.
- The schoolteachers work steadily behind the scenes to facilitate interaction, documenting the process and implementing a practical program that could serve as a model for genuine "Integrated Study*" in schools in communities across the country. It is a program that demonstrates the important role our children's schools can play in building communities for people with dementia in the years ahead.
- The driving force behind the program has been the organization and staff of the facility for the elderly. Their activities offer a model for facilities and staff nationwide that want to pursue exchange and activities with local schools.

2 Day care for people with dementia – the shopping street as springboard for closer community ties

Iki-Iki (vital) day-care service, Hakuaisha Social Welfare Corporation/Osaka Prefecture

Description of activities

Seniors with dementia at Iki-Iki Day-Care Service have become a natural part of the community of the Mitsuya Shotengai shopping street, a kindly and caring neighborhood in Osaka's Yodogawa-ku. Hakuaisha, the social welfare corporation that operates Iki-Iki Day-Care Service, has a history of about 120 years, but Iki-Iki was the first undertaking that took us off the premises and into the community. The impetus came from the passionate commitment of our staff, who wanted to rethink institutional care and find a way to get back to Hakuaisha's basic principle that "the elderly come first." With these goals in mind we opened the center on April 4, 2005. Iki-Iki offers no special recreational activities or other formal programs. Instead, it provides a place outside the home where people with dementia can spend their time normally and naturally. We emphasize and value each aspect of daily life. The big event of the day at Iki-Iki is mealtime. Our motto is, "Decide today's meal today!" Sometimes we all go out to the shopping street and decide the menu together by seeing what the stores have. We also have our seniors do the cooking by consulting with one another. To supplement ordinary contact with the shopkeepers and others on the shopping street, Iki-Iki publishes a newsletter for the merchants and families of people with dementia. We also set up a booth at the summer street festival. In this way the lifestyle of our day-care center helps us fit in naturally as members of the neighborhood.

Positive outcomes

1 SENIORS USING THE CENTER

People at Iki-Iki go actively out onto the shopping street instead of spending all their time indoors. In this way the seniors make acquaintances and develop places with which they are familiar and comfortable. Some seniors who are hard of hearing and not in the habit of conversing have begun greeting the shopkeepers on their own initiative.

2 STAFF

The staff have become more flexible in their thinking and able to approach each person in accordance with his or her individual needs, instead of giving everyone the same cookie-cutter treatment.

3 SHOPKEEPERS, ETC.

There were some shopkeepers on the shopping street who were worried that they would be unable to offer service tailored to seniors. However, when they saw the seniors from Iki-Iki shopping or strolling up and down the shopping street chatting, they gained an appreciation of the importance of this style of service. The Iki-Iki owes its success to the understanding and cooperation of the shopkeepers and others on the shopping street and of community residents.

Reasons for awarding the prize

- As the program has continued, it has been wonderful to see the residents of the community coming to accept as perfectly natural the sight of people with dementia living enjoyable, vital lives within the community.
- In a society that tends to put efficiency above all else, the program demonstrates that even people with dementia can continue to live naturally within the community if they have a relaxed, low-key environment that values each individual and people helping to sustain that environment.
- The program has been implemented in a small corner of the city, but this very element gives it tremendous potential to spread throughout the country.
- The program offers a model that we would like to see adopted in care service providers around the country, as it goes beyond the conventional concepts and systems associated with day care by placing top priority on how the seniors themselves want to spend their time, and by employing staff that are committed to helping people live according to their own preferences and their own pace despite their dementia.

3 Seniors with dementia can be teachers!

School Outside of School (Kosha no nai Gakko; specified nonprofit corporation)/Gifu Prefecture

Description of activities

School Outside of School (Kosha no nai Gakko) carries out a training program in which people learn "genuine life skills" through participation in farm experiences and community life. The name School Outside of School derives from the concept of having the community itself be the schoolhouse in which learning takes place. In this program, seniors, people with dementia, disabled persons, teenagers, children, and even toddlers can become teachers, and the participants learn a great many things while spending time together in an actual living environment. Each hands-on training workshop goes on for three days and two nights. The first day begins with a home stay in a group home or the home of an elderly person in the community. Participants bring cooking ingredients to their home stay destination, and prepare dinner that evening and breakfast the following morning while receiving directions on how to cook it. People with dementia, single seniors, or elderly couples act as the instructors. We pay an instructional fee to the seniors who play this role. The words of the impressed and grateful students are often sufficient reward, but our view is that the fee testifies to the truly useful role these people are playing in society in their job as instructors. Participants rediscover the resources of the people, nature, culture, social services, and industry of their local community and deepen their understanding.

Positive outcomes

1 PARTICIPANTS

Among the "students" was a doctor interested in community health care. He listened to an instructor, a person with dementia, talk about the work he used to do and encourage the doctor, urging him to "Study hard!" "I got a real sense of the inner resources of people with dementia, and I was deeply impressed," the doctor wrote, and he went on to become actively involved in community health care. Questionnaires administered after the overnight workshops indicate that the participants feel they have learned "genuine life skills" from their contact with the instructors and the overnight experience.

2 PEOPLE WITH DEMENTIA

The residents of group home accepted the withdrawn teenager who participated without prejudice and demonstrated their capacity to open his heart to others. The teenager had no time to shut the seniors out before he was chatting freely with them. He went home smiling, with the hosts urging him to stay just a little longer. The capacity of the seniors to accept people just as they are elicited the admiration of everyone, and made them wonder whether dementia gave the seniors a special ability. The seniors themselves performed their role as instructors admirably. Their vitality and enthusiasm sprang from situations in which they were putting their own abilities to use.

Reasons for awarding the prize

- This program not only brings out the potential of people with dementia but teaches us how essential each senior citizen is to our society and what a valuable human resource they represent.
- In the course of "training" by living together, the teenagers learn something from the sight of these enthusiastic, active seniors, gaining a firsthand understanding of the potential of the elderly and how important it is for them to live natural, ordinary lives, and this process is wonderful to behold. People see people with dementia living within the culture and climate of their hometown, and the circle of supporters and sympathizers grows.

- This program leverages the unique culture and climate of a given locale to support people with dementia and build a community.

4 *"Support program for family" Alzheimer's Caregivers Support Workshop – people with dementia are happier when their caregivers are emotionally grounded*

Alzheimer's Association Japan, Aichi Branch/Aichi Prefecture

Description of activities

The Support Program for Family was established to support families that are having problems with caring for their elderly members and to help them to provide the best care they can as soon as possible. The program offers workshops consisting of six sessions, one session per month. Each workshop is attended by a group of about 20 regular members. More than 500 people have enrolled overall. The workshops are led primarily by families with experience in home care. Workshops are divided between periods for gaining knowledge and periods for informal exchange with other caregivers. During the "gaining knowledge" periods, specialists in the medical profession explain the basics of dementia, how to communicate with physicians, and so forth, while other professionals offer advice on care methods and how to make use of formal services. During the "exchange" periods, the caregivers talk with one another, realize that they are not the only ones with such problems, and learn the importance of establishing a care routine that is right for them. We are also working on leadership training to enable anyone to implement this program anywhere in the country; we have already compiled a leadership manual and video.

Positive outcomes

1 PARTICIPANTS

Typical of the feedback we have received are statements like "I gained confidence in my ability to get through any situation. I feel I have grown," and "I met people with all kinds of troubles and realized that I'm not the only one." We have seen many cases where families that began the program looking drawn and overburdened left it with faces expressing relief and optimism. Participants themselves have expressed their desire to continue getting together after the end of a workshop, and in many areas they have begun holding regular get-togethers. In a nearby town, the members of such a group planned and put on a lecture to inform people in the community about dementia, and more than 200 people attended.

2 PEOPLE WITH DEMENTIA

We see many cases in which people with dementia grow calmer as a result of the changes in the way their families relate to them.

3 LOCAL GOVERNMENT

There are indications that program participants in each area are forming a nucleus of community support for caregiver families in cooperation with local government administrators. From a local government's standpoint, these people provide strong and welcome support for dementia care.

Reasons for awarding the prize

- Alzheimer's Association Japan took the lead in creating the Support Program for Family based on years of achievement in this area, and in the course of implementing it has achieved tangible results. Beyond providing support, the association has conducted rigorous monitoring to enhance the program and provide a clear view of its prospects. We believe it offers a concrete model for family support nationwide.
- When family caregivers are emotionally grounded, it leads to improvements in people with dementia. The content of the workshops goes beyond helping families get support and instead places a thoroughgoing emphasis on helping them discover their own ability. In this sense it provides a concrete model that pointing the way for future care.
- Community residents and government offices have assisted in formulating the content and making preparations, and this process has enhanced understanding and support. Along with the support program itself, the approach we have taken to these activities offers lessons for family support efforts going on all around the country.

5 A safety patrol that includes group home residents as community members helping keep children safe

Group Home Mizuhashi House/Toyama Prefecture

Description of activities

In the community where Mizuhashi House is located, a safety patrol has been set up to protect children from crime. Residents of the "group home" are participating in this activity as members of the *Chojukai* (Longevity Society). The impetus for participation came out of the fact that one of the watch stations for the safety patrol proposed by the PTA was within sight of the group home. The route schoolchildren take to and from school coincided with the course that residents of the group home use for their walks. The job of patrol guards is to stand watch at the intersection on their assigned day, wearing a safety patrol armband, starting from the time the children are dismissed from school. Apart from their assigned shifts, the residents of Mizuhashi House also treat their walk time as patrol duty. To help the residents themselves understand that they are performing a useful function and to make the task enjoyable, they wear special *hanten* jackets that they made together with the staff. We have also affixed a "Crime Prevention Patrol" sticker to the car used by the group home and have residents carry out their patrol duties when they get in the car to go shopping, visit the doctor, and so forth.

Positive outcomes

1 PEOPLE WITH DEMENTIA

A sense of purpose and duty about going out on patrol energizes the minds and bodies of the residents, even those who are generally reluctant to go out. In winter, residents are often unwilling to go out in the cold and tend to suffer from lack of exercise as a result, but their determination to go out on patrol has helped solve this problem.

2 GROUP HOME AND COMMUNITY

Recently people from the community recognized residents of the group home when they participated in the community's summer festival and took a snapshot of the occasion for the residents to keep. Thanks to the kindness of community members, residents of the group home are now invited to participate in sports days, school open house presentations, and other school events. Their patrol activities have given them a foothold in the community and allowed them to gradually meld into it. Modest though it may be, we are hopeful that this initiative will spread and that in the future it will become common for people with dementia to act as protectors, not just the protected.

Reasons for awarding the prize

• A wonderful aspect of this program is that it demonstrates, by their actual activities within the community, that people with dementia can be contributors to society and not merely recipients of assistance as kind protectors helping ensure that the children of the community can live there in safety.
• Thanks to this activity, people who had refused to go out can now be seen moving about energetically on their own initiative. In this sense it offers a more advanced model by enabling people to continue being useful to others in their daily lives. The program demonstrates the possibility and the necessity of reconsidering concepts like personal fulfillment and rehabilitation within the context of each patient's life.

- The program demonstrates the possibility for a group home, acting as a base within the community, to send the community the message that we all need to reconsider our hectic way of life.
- The program is a steady, patient undertaking, and its success is the result of the day-to-day efforts of the staff who support the residents in these activities. If group homes throughout Japan would launch efforts of this sort, it would have a positive impact not only on the quality of support for patients but also on the value system of other people in the community.

6 Forest Forum

Forest Forum Steering Committee/Fukuoka Prefecture

Description of activities

The Forest Forum is a newly launched undertaking to give people with dementia, their families, and other community members the opportunity to meet and mingle naturally by spending time together in the natural environment of Yamada Green Park (148.5 hectares) in Kitakyushu city. On the day of the event, 1426 city residents, including 179 people with dementia, gathered to enjoy an autumn day. At the event site, a panel exhibit on dementia was set up and a training course for "dementia supporters", who assist people with dementia and their families in the communities, held to enhance participants' accurate understanding of dementia. Under a blue sky, participants freely joined in such group activities as woodland hikes, paper making, open-air nursing care classes, and a free market, according to their preferences. From the planning stages people from all sectors cooperated in putting on the Forest Forum, including environmental volunteers, welfare volunteers, ordinary citizens, and people from non-profit organizations, schools, business, and government. Through this they were able to discover a shared perspective on "community building" that transcends their own sectors. We are now working on compiling a manual that will make it possible to launch a similar undertaking in any community. The manual will contain in a compact format the information and materials needed to make the organization of such an event practical in other communities.

Positive outcomes

1 PEOPLE WITH DEMENTIA

At the event itself many people told us that ordinarily blank-faced seniors began smiling as they came in contact with nature and with other people. The patients themselves offered a variety of positive comments, remarking, "The scenery here is so peaceful. And the air smells nice, too." Everyone was amazed at the forest's "healing powers," and at the end of the day not only the people with dementia but the other participants as well felt the forest had given some of its vitality to them.

2 PARTICIPANTS, RESIDENTS

Volunteers in the environmental and welfare fields were able to share their know-how and collaborate rather than pigeon-holing dementia as a nursing or welfare issue. As a result, environmental volunteers, welfare volunteers, ordinary citizens, and people from nonprofits, schools, businesses, and government agencies brought together what they had to offer and did what came naturally to them, and the event proceeded smoothly. We received requests to extend the event to a wider range of sites in the city as well. At the Forest Forum we made maximum use of people's accustomed activities and the community's resources. The undertaking made everyone realize that community resources can be found everywhere without doing anything special.

Reasons for awarding the prize

- The program is unique in that an environmental not for profit organization (NPO) worked together with local government to hold it, escaping from the confines of the standard social welfare model, and in the way it made use of a "forest" within an urban community.
- It was wonderful to see the way natural understanding and interaction with people with dementia developed and the way participants brought out each another's strengths as people of all sorts—with dementia and without, adults, students, and small children—met in the "forest" and felt its power together. We believe that in this way community building will advance, slowly but surely.
- The program offers something new in its collaborative approach, bringing together the know-how of administrators, professionals, and volunteers from the environmental and welfare sectors.
- The program has nurtured broader partnerships between different administrative offices and agencies, and it has contributed to administrators' understanding of people with dementia and of the importance of community building to support such people. In this sense it offers a model for local administration throughout the country.

7 Community advocacy for people with dementia

Iga City Council of Social Welfare/Mie Prefecture

Description of activities

Iga City Council of Social Welfare is at work on a comprehensive community-wide program enlisting ordinary citizens to protect the civil and human rights of people with dementia. The program comprises the following specific undertakings.

- Development of a community care system (from 1985);
- Organization of a caregivers association (from 1990);

- Community welfare rights advocacy program (from 2000);
- Respite care program (from 2003);
- Program to fight unscrupulous business practices (from 2004);
- Iga City Counseling Network (from 2004);
- Welfare Guardianship Support Center (from 2006).

A particularly urgent issue was the steady rise in reports of unscrupulous business practices, which seemed to be increasing faster than authorities' ability to uncover and deal with them. To address this problem, we decided to hold an Iga Fraud Busters Training Workshop predicated on the concept of "stamping out fraud through citizen participation." Attorneys, staff from the Consumer Affairs Center, and others taught a series of seven classes attended by 36 citizens. In fiscal 2006, the program was able to prevent unscrupulous business transactions totaling approximately ¥30 million. By leveraging the power of ordinary citizens, we are working to build a community where people with dementia can live in safety and security.

Positive outcomes

Through its wide-ranging efforts, the Iga City Council of Social Welfare has helped nurture within the community a growing network of individual citizens and groups that understand and support people with dementia. If enough citizens take an interest in the rights of people with dementia and related issues and in looking after their welfare, unscrupulous operators will not be able to take advantage of them. The Fraud Busters perform the following functions:

1   uncovering unscrupulous business practices and directing victims to counseling services
2   helping people exercise their right to a cooling-off period [for purchases]
3   communicating information on previous cases of unscrupulous business practices
4   working as a team to defeat fraudulent sales techniques and others.

In addition, by participating in the process of solving the problems faced by people with dementia and their families, citizens learn to sympathize with the circumstances and predicaments in which such people find themselves and share in their worries, their joys, and their sorrows. It is also a program that allows people to start thinking early about how they would like things to be if this should happen to them. As a growing number of citizens understand and relate to people with dementia and as various measures are undertaken on their behalf, we take a giant step toward becoming a community where people can continue to live in safety and security even if afflicted with dementia.

Reasons for awarding the prize

- For a community to be "dementia friendly," it is important to take measures against unscrupulous business practices and enhance our "adult guardianship." This program is involved in ongoing, realistic efforts, such as training of citizen supporters and the Fellowship Salon, that put the power of private citizens to work with positive results.
- Through wide-ranging activities, the program is instilling in citizens a perspective that asks, "What can be done to protect the rights of people with dementia?" To ensure that people with dementia can live in security, both the idea and the reality of rights advocacy are critical. In this sense the program can provide hints for other communities and a wide range of other activities.
- Social welfare councils exist in communities throughout Japan. This program makes use of the special character of a social welfare council and as such can serve as a reference for similar undertakings around the country.

8 Expanding the "Omuta City wandering-senior safety network" through simulation drills

Hayame-Minami Human Kindness Network/Fukuoka Prefecture

Description of activities

Since 2004, an annual "wandering-senior simulation drill" has been carried out under the leadership of the Hayame-Minami Human Kindness Network. In 2006, the drill was carried out with wide-ranging cooperation from community members (about 200 participants representing about 100 groups), including representatives from the police and fire departments, city hall, the Association of Nursing Care Services, local welfare and child-welfare commissioners, the Taxi Association, construction firms, construction firms, and local schools. Hayame-Minami Human Kindness Network began with a grassroots idea for building a network based on immediate neighborhood ties and a community gathering place. After a series of discussions among the community residents of Hayame-Minami School District, the network was formally launched in February 2004 as an organization through which community volunteers could act in concert. On the day of the drill, a community member, who had taken the "dementia supporter" training course, gently guided the person playing the role of a wandering and exhausted person with dementia back to safety. In 2006, prior to the drill, a training course for "dementia supporters" was held for people in the police and fire departments, local construction firms, and so forth, helping to deepen understanding in the community.

Positive outcomes

1 RESIDENTS OF HAYAME-MINAMI DISTRICT

Today, if an individual wanders off and disappears somewhere in the city of Omuta, the Hayame-Minami Human Kindness Network notifies approximately 70 residents, shops, and other volunteers in the Hayame-Minami district, and the residents begin investigating and keeping watch in their immediate neighborhood. The system also ensures that any sighting or other information is promptly reported back. Meanwhile, the Omuta Police Department's existing SOS Network has improved the speed and mobility of its city-wide response. In this way, the wandering-senior simulation drill has yielded very positive results. The drills have helped deepen citizens' understanding of people with dementia, encouraged them to approach and talk to any senior they find wandering, and have fostered a network in which residents look after one another.

2 THE CITY OF OMUTA

There is now a common information sheet for the entire city of Omuta, which is continually being put to use. Each year there are approximately 120 cases of missing persons, and the network is mobilized for about 20 of those cases. Unfortunately, each year one or two such cases have ended in the death of the person. At the time of writing, there had been no deaths since October 2006.

Reasons for awarding the prize

- Through this unique "wandering-senior simulation drill" program, practical measures have been taken to address the serious problem of people with dementia wandering off and disappearing. The program has been a factor behind the enhanced efficacy of the SOS Network established to respond "when the unexpected happens."
- The program has contributed to concrete community-wide network building embracing a wide range of individuals and organizations. The development, through the power of community networking, of a community where people with dementia can be safe even if they should wander away, offers a nationwide model for the future. Through the simulation drill, understanding toward people with dementia has deepened, and the awareness of the police concerning this issue has improved.
- The program has begun to spread beyond the city of Omuta to other municipalities. This is important for the improvement of support for wandering seniors, in which wide-area response is essential.
- The program involves a two-pronged effort: spreading understanding among community residents on the one hand, and implementing concrete, practical steps to protect people with dementia on the other.

- Government and citizens are thinking and acting together. This aspect of community building through the united efforts of the public and private sector also provides a model for the nation.

Note

* The "Period for Integrated Study" aims at helping children develop capability and ability to discover problems by themselves and solve those problems properly. (National Curriculum Standards Reform for Elementary School, Ministry of Education, 1998).

Further information

Please visit: www.ninchisho100.net/english/index.html.

10 Discovering options

An Australian initiative in the care of the dying

Helen-Anne Manion, Gerard Manion and Kathleen Dansie

The Australian background

HOME Hospice was founded in Australia in 1980 by Dr Helen-Anne Manion, a GP and subsequently palliative care specialist, and Gerard Manion, a cancer counsellor, and now functions as a charitable organisation operating in several parts of that country. It originated from a request by a patient attending Gerard Manion's Cancer Care programme. Knowing his death was imminent, the patient asked for help to remain at home, to be able to die supported by the love of family in the comfort of familiar surroundings. This request was the first of many. Dr Manion had observed no lack of friends visiting the homes of the dying but noticed that the principal carers often had such friends added to their already stressful workload (*'you'll have a cuppa with us? No, no, no problem at all! Just sit there and I'll make it – tea or coffee for you?'*). Loving friends and caring neighbours wished to demonstrate their concern; how could this be used to assist principal carers in their work of looking after the dying, where they belonged, in their own homes?

For its development in Australia, the founders of HOME Hospice wished to advance three aspects of palliative care. The first was that a dying person, who wanted it, should be enabled to remain at home. The second was to support the role of the carer, for all too often the loving carer sacrificed self in trying to meet the needs of the dying. Often there were drastic repercussions for one who provided sole care, yet received little or no support themselves (Briggs and Fisher 2000; Aoun 2004). Finally, the founding team believed that friends and neighbours could undertake essential roles, compassionately serving the carer so that person was able to focus more completely on the needs of the dying relation.

The emphasis on home (in upper case) as the setting, distinguishes HOME Hospice from institutions offering palliative care, such as a hospice. While the word 'hospice' is derived from Latin and indicates both host and guest (Hanks *et al.* 1986), by its very nature as an institution it cannot offer the freedom of movement to friends and family over every 24 hours, nor the sense of belonging that can be achieved in a person's home. HOME Hospice focuses on the crucial role of the dying person's carer. Manion developed her role as a mentor for carers and the founders trained others to take on this role (see Figure 10.1).

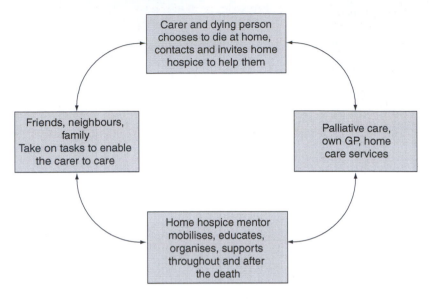

Figure 10.1 HOME Hospice relationship model.

With simple organisational structures in place, practical needs could be rostered between friends and relations. This step conserved the time and energies of the carer. It met the need of community membership too, in that it suggested a pathway for action for individuals in a compassionate society. In the past century or so, dying had become a realm in which community had little or, increasingly, no place, and where the appearance of friends and neighbours was restricted to attendance at the funeral. Structures developed by HOME Hospice 're-discovered' past customs, when the personal community (family, friends, neighbours) bonded closely together, to sustain the carer and the immediate family.

In the past, dying at home was accepted as the norm: it was free, personal and arguably enhanced family bonding (Whitelaw 2005). Evidence gathered over the past 28 years from the work of HOME Hospice in Australia demonstrates multiple benefits from the home based approach. Most importantly, the dying person, lovingly cared for in their own environment, is saved from loneliness and the countless indignities of institutional care, where they would have no control over process and implementation of that process. Carer Christine, who cared for her mother for five weeks before she passed away in their home stated in an interview, '*directed and guided by HOME Hospice it is possible to have quality of life at home throughout the dying journey*' (Woods 1997). Sid, diagnosed with a terminal illness, wanted to remain in his home and contacted HOME Hospice for help for his wife, who was his carer, after reading an advertisement in the local newspaper. Sid said, '*I want this help for Dorothy so that we can stay in our home with our kids right to the end*.' (HOME Hospice 1993–2009).

Significantly, despite the foreseen conclusion of the task, the carer also tends to rejoice, having achieved a difficult and demanding goal, well supported by family and community. Susie, exclaimed, *'the best thing I've ever done'* (Blacker 2001) after the death of her mother, whom she cared for in her home between February and April 2001. *'I've done it'*, Laurie, who cared for his wife and *'I'm so glad that I did this'*, Marg, after caring for her mother: comments from carers recorded by HOME Hospice Mentors (HHM) in their evaluation and files (HOME Hospice 1993–2009). Carer Christine also stated in an interview, *'it is hard to believe that such a tragedy could have such a good outcome'* (Woods 1997). In 1998, Trish who cared for her dying father stated just after his death, *'I've never had children but I feel as though I've just given birth'* (HOME Hospice 1993–2009).

The family's personal community were found to exhibit closer bonding as stated by numerous carers. Bob, who cared for his wife in their home said, *'when you [HHM] first called our friends and neighbours and invited them to a gathering, I couldn't imagine how this could happen but now those same friends and neighbours have gone beyond just friendship. There's a powerful bond. They've become family'* (ibid.). Community members referred to how their previously held views and fears about being close to a dying person had been replaced with a sense of confidence, a sense that they knew how to approach the person, as well as help the carer (ibid.). They spoke of appreciation that they had been needed, that they felt wanted and that they believed there was a definite place for them, mostly an unobtrusive place, but one which filled many requirements (ibid.). In 1997, Norm, a caring neighbour, took on tasks to help care for his neighbour Marg who was carer for her dying mother Vera. Norm delivered the eulogy at Vera's funeral and said, *'HOME Hospice has profoundly influenced the way I view life from now on'* (ibid.).

The HHM is invited by the carer. Carer Christine explained in an interview, *'HOME Hospice won't just go in. You have to want them and invite them first'* (Woods 1997). The HHM presents to the carer and family as a knowledgeable friend, to empower, not to do what community is there to do, but to empower and enable carer, family and community to do their respective roles. The HHM will provide the carer with HH educational booklets (Manion and Manion 1997a, 1997b, 1997c) to help the carer know how to care, what to expect, ensure self care and to live well while caring for the dying loved one. Working alongside HOME Hospice and focusing on the patient is the medical, nursing, palliative care team, and home care services each complementing the other. The HHM's role is to mobilise, motivate and direct community in its care and support for the carer. Likewise, the friends and neighbours are not there to do what the carer is to do, that is to care for the dying loved one. They are empowered to care for the carer. Carer Martin, said after the death of his wife in their home, *'my neighbours freed up my time so that I could spend more time with Cheryl'* (HOME Hospice Inc. Files 1993–2009).

Support for the Australian research into HOME Hospice is becoming more widespread. Kellehear's work on health promoting palliative care and the vital input of community participation in end of life care has attracted considerable attention (1999, 2005). He argues that the present medical model of palliative care, largely based around symptom management, is no longer satisfactory. This medicalised, institutionalised model should be infused by one that not only recognises the need for holistic care of the dying person, but equally involves community participation at all levels in designing their own ways to care for one another (Sallnow *et al.* 2009). Symptom management is vital but the empowering of the dying person's carer and personal community, is of even greater consequence (Manion H.-A *et al.* 2009).

The African experiment

Phase one: 2003

In 2001, the Australian experience with HOME Hospice was shared by Dr Manion with personnel in palliative care and public health fields in Switzerland and the USA (The World Health Organization, Open Society Institute; World Bank Human Development Network). Expressions of support for the HOME Hospice philosophy were universal. HOME Hospice was seen as a programme intimately involving family, friends and neighbours in end of life care. The emphasis on engagement of the dying person's 'personal community' attracted the attention of medical personnel, who suggested that it could be applied to countries in southern Africa where HIV/AIDS are devastating numerous communities.

The question of how this could be funded was paramount. HOME Hospice Australia has functioned for most of its life on donations and contributions from private donors, many of whom experienced HOME Hospice as part of the personal community of the carer and dying loved one. Funds are also raised through the fundraising activities by HOME Hospice Inc. members, the founder's local church groups and service clubs, and Rotary Foundation International. Most work was done on a voluntary basis by the carer and patient's 'personal community' as was that of the founders. Dr Manion succeeded in interesting Rotary Foundation International (RFI) in the possibility of the HOME Hospice Program being implemented in selected communities in some countries of southern Africa. In 2003, Manion, another medical doctor and an associate were awarded funds by the RFI to travel to South Africa, Swaziland and Botswana to assess the viability of the application of the philosophy and principles of HOME Hospice to communities there.

What had been learnt from preparatory reading about the health care situation in many states in Africa was confirmed when the Rotary team visited Home Based Care (HBC) services in both rural and urban settings in southern Africa. The HBC services provided care for those suffering with HIV/AIDS, tuberculosis and many other diseases. Additionally they observed and evaluated programmes for AIDS orphans, and palliative care programmes for the dying offered in hospices. People living with HIV/AIDS faced a myriad of problems. In addition to endemic poverty and its associated problems of insufficient and/or inappropriate ill-nourishing foods and unsafe water supplies, some belief systems impacted disproportionately on people living with HIV/AIDS. These included beliefs that the disease was the result of witchcraft – a belief largely unchallenged by both government and health authorities. Some people in high office even claimed that there was no such disease at all. The former President of South Africa, Thabo Mbeke, stated this in 1999 (van Rijn, 2006). Superstition and fear frequently meant that sufferers of HIV/AIDS were abandoned to die without medical or palliative care.

The Rotary team found that HIV/AIDS in southern Africa carried a stigma with it, as it has in many parts of our world, a stigma moreover, which tended to increase the discrimination experienced by sufferers. Communities were further fractured as a result. Breakdown of community had been in evidence for many years, and times of forced labour migration to find work and apartheid had all exacerbated this. Often, too often, the only persons left to care for the dying were children, some as young as seven. And for them, or a carer of any age, there was virtually no support.

While the Rotary team applauded the work effected through the HBC programmes, they felt that the HOME Hospice approach would address the needs of the carer and would help engage community members, possibly leading to an increase in the social cohesiveness of a local community. As they travelled through South Africa, Swaziland and Botswana, the Rotary team addressed a variety of audiences, and presented their ideas about the value of the HOME Hospice philosophy in palliative care work. As a result of one such meeting, the AIDS Program Coordinator for the Diocese of Tzaneen, in the Limpopo Province of South Africa, asked team members to establish HOME Hospice throughout their Diocese. Training of personnel so that there would be a focus in palliative care on both the carer and the patient was wanted and this resulted in the 2004 and 2006 visits of HOME Hospice trainers.

Phase two: 2004

Back in Australia, HOME Hospice members Dr Manion, Gerard Manion and Kathleen Dansie had numerous meetings and workshops over eight months (January-August 2004) to review, evaluate and adapt the existing Australian HH 'Training Manual for Mentors' and 'Notes for Carers' (Manion and Manion 1997a, 1997b) in order to meet conditions in Tzaneen. Communication sessions were held with the AIDS Program Coordinator for the Diocese of Tzaneen via email and phone conferencing to establish aims and objectives, programme content, and environment and cultural orientation. Information in the already existing manuals was simplified into flow charts. To address language barriers, pictorial illustrations were used. The African HOME Hospice Program was totally aligned with the mission statement of the organisation: 'the vision of HOME Hospice is a world in which families and their communities are empowered to regain their proper role in the care of their terminally ill loved ones.' The African programme had a three fold emphasis:

a   a focus on the needs of and support for the carer;
b   a focus on engaging personal community members to provide that support;
c   a focus on maintaining the dignity of all involved in the palliative care process.

Training materials were produced in Australia for trialling. These detailed a process through which all trainees would pass and provided much of the basis for current and follow-up action research. In this first iteration the materials were used in the Diocese of Tzaneen, which covers approximately 51,000 square kilometres in the Limpopo Province and extends to the Zimbabwe border. The three member HOME Hospice team divided the training between them. Dr Manion dealt with 'the what' – what HOME Hospice does; Gerard Manion with 'the why' – the philosophy and beliefs underlying HOME Hospice; and Kathleen Dansie with 'the how' – how to work with the carers, dying and those grieving.

Over the period of one month (September 2004), the trainers worked with 100 African volunteers, known as HOME Hospice Facilitators (HHFs) at Mootketsi. Volunteers travelled great distances, often in harsh circumstances, to train in the HOME Hospice Program (HHP) so they could return to their villages and implement its practices. These were new and challenging experiences for everyone involved – the facilitators and the training team.

The philosophy and practices of HOME Hospice were presented to the HHFs in a series of modules. HOME Hospice's own training materials (Manion and Manion 1997a, 1997b and 1997c) were the basis of these. Dr Manion's booklet on Free Medicines (Manion H.-A. 2006) was also a key source and adapted for African conditions and scenes. The Australian version of this had been in use for over 15 years. Illustrations and drawings explained the many ways by which pain and discomfort can be relieved. The pictorial 'Free Medicines' book was made available for distribution to carers in 2006. Additional flow charts and information sheets were prepared and formed the basis of key sessions.

Preliminary sessions covered concepts about complementary work; HHFs would work alongside and in addition to Home Based Carers. They have different roles but are complementary in creating optimum conditions for the dying. HHFs were to understand that their work was in partnership with that of others; research arising from this initial programme would show how best to devise ways HOME Hospice could be most useful in the Tzaneen situation. The conditions set by HOME Hospice were clarified: all care was free, given by volunteers in the dying person's home. A holistic approach was to be taken towards the sick person's needs – needs of body, mind and spirit, not just needs prompted by physical diseases. The HHFs would learn that the key to helping was the welfare of the carer; help from friends and neighbours was indispensable.

Some formal education giving greater knowledge and understanding about HIV/AIDS was seen as necessary to help to counter superstition. Dr Manion, the palliative care specialist on the team, used visuals in order to teach the cause and progression of the disease. Follow-up discussions helped to establish confidence and knowledge in the trainees, reducing or eliminating fears and stigmas. During a role play session, an HHF confidently allayed a carer's fear of people discovering that there was a sick person with AIDS in their home (HOME Hospice 2006).

The training programme presented five distinct phases of learning. How to make contact with the carer and the first visit with them was an initial area of learning. Ideally an introductory visit to the home of the sick person, which followed on a specific invitation, would be made in company with the HBC, so all concerned could see how the HOME Hospice structure could work with existing carers and yet offer more. HHFs were trained (videos, slides, discussions, workshops) in explaining how to introduce themselves and what they could offer. An emphasis was placed on the HOME Hospice's focus on the carer, so the HHFs would understand the difference between HOME Hospice and HBC – which focused on the patient's physical needs. The HHF would be in the home of the dying person as a knowledgeable friend, supporting and organising additional help.

The first visit was seen as the time to observe, ask, learn and record. Observation of living conditions would guide the HHF in knowing what kind of help may be needed. The age of the primary carer would be noted – so many are children and their needs would be different from those of an adult carer. The HHF would enquire about what the family wanted in all three areas of physical, mental and spiritual needs. Preparatory questions about what may happen after death could be generated, and on leaving, the HHF would assure the primary carer that there would be time to discuss all these aspects and any others on the subsequent visit. Brief notes written now were written up in detail on returning to the home base.

The awareness and first visit training session were followed by what HOME Hospice considers to be the most important section in its programme: The Gathering. This means the gathering together of any friends, neighbours, relations or others who will volunteer to assist the primary carer. The HOME Hospice facilitator was trained to list what jobs needed to be done and to talk with the family about any persons living nearby who may have offered help. Then the HHF would approach village members explaining the needs and asking for help. A roster would be developed. This was time consuming but extremely worthwhile. These helpers represent the carer's personal community; they need to know how much they are appreciated, and how much they can bond together as a team to offer the dignity of service.

The remaining two training sessions involved what to do on follow-up visits and at the time of death; how to help a dying loved one; the signs that death may be near and how to comfort the grieving.

Research findings from phase two

Evaluation sheets were issued at the beginning of each HH training session. A multilingual trainee assisted with interpreting questions and answers. The HH team read the evaluations, noted comments and promptly addressed any issues.

The HH team continued to hold meetings with the AIDS Program Coordinator for the Diocese of Tzaneen and her assistants to liaise and gauge the value of the programme. Research included comments and conversations from evaluations and formal and informal meetings (Cohen and Manion 1994).

In the Tzaneen Diocese, a HBC programme had been developed and functioned through their Kurisanani administrative centre in Tzaneen. It offered palliative care in the home without medication as this was unavailable. The HOME Hospice team were unaware that the majority of the 100 new trainees had been selected from this pre-existing palliative care group. HBC organisers at Kurisanani sent out flyers and invitations to HBC volunteers, palliative care workers and health clinics throughout the Tzaneen Diocese. Consequently, the trainees offered HOME Hospice a great advantage in that, as HBCs, they already had access to carers and patients through their previous home visiting. However, the trainees were asked to alter their primary perspective; they were, with HOME Hospice, to have their primary focus on the carer rather than on care of the patient.

Some 90 per cent of the trainees were Christian and were drawn from village populations. Most experienced poverty; some were also HIV positive. Their village backgrounds facilitated their forming 'Gathering' sessions and about a quarter of the trainees did this (see Appendix 6 for details of the questionnaire). Their remarks from evaluation forms distributed at the beginning of each training session indicate that they realised the significance of their focus on the carer and saw the difference between that and HBC's focus solely on a patient's physical needs.

> *Teaching about it being so important to take care of our sick ones in their own homes with their family, friends and neighbours, rather than in hospitals with people (nurses) they don't know.*
>
> (HOME Hospice Trainee Joyce 2004)

Trainees found the follow-up workshops and open forums valuable. There they were encouraged to speak openly about issues of concern and three areas were quickly identified: breaking down the barriers of fear and stigma, educating for social change and how to restore dignity and encourage friendship amongst all who were involved in primary care in a village setting. The question of stigma was a key one. Such is the overwhelming fear of disclosure, research from this visit showed that only 29 per cent of the carers disclosed they were helping patients dying with HIV/AIDS. As Marcus reported:

> ... their illness (HIV/AIDS) sends shock waves into a social web that has as its epicentre their immediate family, but which extends to more distant relatives, friends, neighbours, colleagues and social acquaintances ... the very scale of the micro social shocks has mezzo and macro impacts that require a level of social mobilization that extends well beyond the particular circumstances and experiences of the individual who is diagnosed as HIV+.
>
> (Marcus 2002)

It was decided to appoint a local coordinator to promote the availability of HOME Hospice in parishes and village clusters in Tzaneen, Modjajiskloof, Makhado, Phalaborwa, Malamulele and Ofcolaco. Lutendo, a trainee, was multilingual and developed a thorough understanding of and enthusiasm for the HH programme. As an energetic and respected leader, Lutendo became the appointed African Program Coordinator, was given many roles, but primarily was to meet with HHFs in six parishes where the programme was operating and was to generate teaching materials for the HHFs from what had already been developed by the Australian team. Support from Australia was assured.

Phase three: 2006

The overarching aims of this next visit to Africa were to refresh trainees and to accompany them in their work in the villages. To achieve this, the HOME Hospice team was funded by private donors and Caritas Australia. The health situation in Tzaneen remained dire. The Tzaneen Diocese had introduced anti-retroviral treatment but could offer it to only a limited number of patients, approximately 200 in 2006 (O'Leary 2009), both due to the fear patients had of disclosing their disease and the lack of funding for the drugs. Clinics and hospitals failed to keep pace with the pandemic and those with HIV/AIDS were frequently turned away from institutions despite having travelled long distances to seek help. Traditional healers, Sangomas, were still popular and used by some 14 per cent of the people (HH survey questionnaire 2006).

The Sisters in the Tzaneen Diocese had continued their work with the Kurisanani trained HBCs and the numbers of children and families needing their support had continued to rise. Patients too weak to access local clinics depended on the HBCs for supplies. There had been no further development of palliative care in the region and both the medical needs and the medical structures remained unchanged.

The HH team of Dr Manion, Gerard Manion and Kathleen Dansie worked from October 2005 to April 2006 in Australia to develop a four-day training programme to deliver at three different sites. As far as possible, training was implemented within close proximity to the parish in which HHFs were working – a total of 13 parishes and 33 villages. Fifty-one trainees took part. Criteria for selection was that they had attended the 2004 training programme and were able to bring their manuals, issued in 2004, to the 2006 training. The emphasis was on melding the roles of HBCs with that of HHFs. Day 1 of the programme involved the cultural courtesy of meeting with the chief to inform about HH and to ascertain approval to visit the carers and their dying loved one in their village home with HHFs on Day 4 of the training programme.

Many different strategies were employed to ensure all trainees were as comfortable as possible with their learning. Small group discussions were found to assist analysis and to enhance inclusiveness. The majority of trainees were women (85 per cent) and there were many discussions about the roles of women in African society (see Figure 10.2). Empowering of women in this culture,

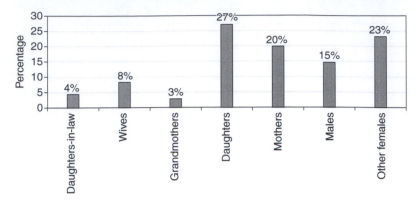

Figure 10.2 Relationship of carers to patients.

together with education and awareness, could have a significant impact on stemming the AIDS pandemic (Dowling 2002).

Some of the male trainees were reluctant to take on tasks they considered to be women's work and educational sessions were designed to help overcome this (in one family a 12-year-old brother did not want to learn how to help the carer because, he said, '*it is a girl thing*'). Additional flow charts and focused role plays, particularly those about visiting a carer and the patient, comprised a significant part of the training as, in this phase, trainees undertook visits to villages and homes.

Semi-structured interviews were used to gauge the appropriateness, effectiveness and value of the training programme. Openness and friendship between trainees and trainers were encouraged. Responses were positive: '*HHFs are needed to help and teach people to help others so that the situation is better*' Edwin (HOME Hospice 2006). Trainees enjoyed learning simple techniques, such as foot massage and breathing for relaxation to relieve stress and pain. These arts proved useful as breaks in the packed training days but their real intent was that this knowledge was to be passed on to the carers for the benefit of both the carer and their dying loved one.

HHFs were shown how to encourage children to share in the grieving process and how to deal with their loss. HOME Hospice research from the Trainee Survey (Dansie 2006) showed that 19 per cent of carers were aged between 11 and 20 (see Figure 10.3). As one 13-year old wrote in the survey questionnaire, '*as a child it's hard to take care of a sick person and I felt it was all too much for me. But when HOME Hospice came in things started to change and I felt at ease.*'

An open forum was held with the trainees to discuss the increasing involvement of children as caregivers and the need to support them, despite some cultural inhibitions regarding grief where children are often excluded from being a part of the dying and death of a love one. They are often excluded from information and from taking part in the funeral (Marcus 2002; Martin 2004).

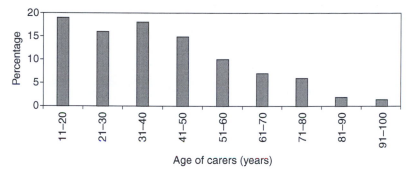

Figure 10.3 Age of carers.

Finally, the question of human contact was covered. In 2004, the HOME Hospice team had observed how terminally ill patients were deprived of the warmth of human contact. This often involved their carers, such was their fear of HIV/AIDS. As a way of trying to overcome the villager's fear of venturing close to HIV patients, Dansie thought of teaching the villagers to knit. With a supply of brightly coloured wool and needles donated in Australia, the team began teaching the HHFs to knit. In turn, they would teach the carers of AIDS patients, attracting others in the village to join them. It was thought this may help solve the problem of the isolation of the carer. The HOME Hospice team constantly emphasised the importance of reviving a sense of community, greatly damaged by forced migrations, poverty and loss of morale. Training sessions around the knitting led to discussions about how to help community cohesion as well as how to knit blankets!

Every training session was videoed by cinematographer Anthony Manion, who accompanied the team. As the films captured gestures, expressions, the environment and, to some degree, the atmosphere, they became, when edited, an ongoing educational resource for HHF trainees. At the end of the six-week training period, all the trained HHFs gathered for a further two-day workshop, to reinforce core learning and to comment upon and finalise planning to sustain the HHP throughout the Diocese. It was decided that Lutendo, the appointed coordinator for the Project, was to plan and conduct monthly meetings for all HHFs as well as being available for advice and support. She was to liaise with Dansie, the Australian Project Manager, and the local parish coordinators to assist with the distribution of materials and wool arriving from Australia.

These monthly meetings were designed to be opportunities for further training, using the video footage for ongoing analysis of needs, wants and concerns. There would be times for socialising and de-briefing as well. Survey questionnaires would be gathered and forwarded to the Australian Project Manager for ongoing action research, as were the reports from the monthly meetings. An agreement had been reached between Caritas, Australia and the Tzaneen Diocese over funding for attendance at the monthly meetings so that the HHP could be sustained. Unfortunately, at the end of 2006 Lutendo, the Tzaneen Diocese Project Coordinator, resigned from her position for personal reasons. As the sole supporter of her family, she was forced to take a higher paying position.

Evaluation of project

A survey questionnaire was the chief research tool used following the 2006 visit (Appendix 6). Questions were asked about the primary carer, the patient, and the HHF. Included in these questions was information about relationships, children, chief concerns of patients and others and support being offered by whom to whom. Questionnaires were returned to Australia and preliminary analysis undertaken. Of particular concern in analysing the raw data was the need to understand the impact of the HHP in the African village settings, its effects on carers, families, patients and on the HHFs, in order to be able to separate our achievements to date against probable future needs.

Findings

On the understanding of the core teachings of HOME Hospice:

> *My sister could not admit her illness, but with HH she can, and is happier.*

> *I encouraged him to call the neighbours and relatives.*

> *I talked to the neighbours and told them that they can help the Carer so that she would not be stressed.*

And during an open forum:

> *Many people must be trained to be HHFs to help people.*

On the support of the carer

> *Our neighbours turned out to be our supporters*

> *HH helped this family situation because the Carer felt we were helping even though it was not easy within our culture for an old age person to accept help.*

On the Free Medicine book

> *After using the 'Free Medicine' book the Carer found it easier to look after her mother.*

> *. . . it [Free Medicine book] removed stress from the family*

On the use of knitting as a device to assist village cohesion

The knitting groups proved to be helpful in several ways. Not only did they assist gathering people together:

> *This knitting project will be helpful to my mother because when I am at school my mother will keep on doing this blanket which will take off the stress. She is happy because she is contributing something to her family.*

> *I support and encourage this blanket making project. My grandchild is now helped and accepted by her neighbours. HOME Hospice Facilitators take their time to sit down with them and teach them how to knit.*

> *Because they could get some wool, the neighbours came to the Gathering. It was a happy situation because then they wanted to help the Carer.*

Core teachings were also instrumental in helping overcome fear of closeness to the dying

> *We are challenged to accept the whole person. AIDS is not the responsibility of the infected/affected alone, but also of the community. Pastoral challenges are to accept, restore dignity and to make people feel at home and part of our community.*
>
> Sr Tshifhiwa Munhedzi (Rule and Melele 2004)

Reflections on HOME Hospice as a programme, revised for implementation in selected African countries

HOME Hospice did translate well to African conditions. Its structure worked. It trained 100 HHFs to mobilise the carers' communities in support of carers and families of those dying at home. One report, sent from Nzhelele in May 2006, said:

> *HOME Hospice is making a lot of difference to the people's life. It solves many problems between carers and patients ... Families, neighbours and community are accepting this HH. They said they were very happy with this knitting project ... and very happy with the Free Medicines book because it helps them when the patient is in a bad condition. All HHFs are doing their work and teaching the Carers. All are interested.*

Challenges of the project

1   Before leaving Australia, members of the Australian HOME Hospice team, having thoroughly researched the situation in Africa, believed they understood the enormity of the AIDS problem, and its deadly consequences in

Africa. Coming to close quarters with the reality, seeing the ravages of the disease in individuals and getting some idea of the dimensions of the pandemic was unsettling, to say the least. At the same time, the team was awed by the way in which people bore the pain and indignity of such suffering.

What compounded the problem was the widespread belief that the cause of HIV/AIDS was understood to be a matter of witchcraft. This was further aggravated by government misinformation denying the very existence of the problem as a matter of illness. In the face of that thinking, HOME Hospice wondered how they could meet the challenge of teaching whole communities the truth about HIV/AIDS to enable them to overcome the fear and superstition which kept them from involvement with those dying victims.

2   Language differences presented some difficulties. HHF trainees were drawn from communities whose first languages were Tsonga, Venda and Zulu. HOME Hospice had made spoken and written English a pre-requisite for selection, but still found some variation in proficiency. Many had difficulty communicating abstract thinking or expressing their feelings. The hypothetical often presented a problem.

3   Any programme which is based on volunteers needs to have a flexible approach towards schedules and changes. The HOME Hospice team was at times required to change schedules without notice, to learn to improvise, and always to be flexible. Despite natural and human made obstructions, the trainees were dedicated, energetic and, above all, compassionate.

4   The resources of all concerned were limited. One effect of this was that the organisations could not increase a salary in order to keep the appointed coordinator. Her loss led to the demise of the programme. There is a message here about reliance on one key person when effecting change. Succession planning is needed in the initial stages of change (Fullan 1993).

By contrast there was much to offset the challenges. What members of the HOME Hospice team saw so happily sustained was the spirit and the spirituality of the people. Trainee HHFs remained strong and hopeful. In the face of suffering and poverty, team members met carers, dying AIDS victims, even their children valiantly caring for them, showing love, patience and character in the midst of tragedy. Spontaneous outbursts of singing together in harmony, evidence of joy and an indomitable spirit became unsurprising. HOME Hospice team members came away with feelings of fellowship, high regard and admiration. The words of the famous song 'We will overcome' were sung often during training and serve to capture the sentiment of people showing tremendous courage in adversity.

Acknowledgements

Jennifer Burnley MA Hons., BA Hons., Dip. Tchg., Dip. L. AM.ST., Dip. R.E.
Anthony Manion, Cinematographer.

References

Aoun, S. (ed.) (2004) *The hardest thing I have ever done: the social impact of caring for terminally ill people in Australia: full report of the National Inquiry into the social impact of caring for terminally ill people incorporating a literature review and analysis of public submissions*, Palliative Care Australia, Australia.

Blacker, S. (2001) *With HOME Hospice, Caring is not a health hazard: interview with Suzie*, [DVD], HOME Hospice Inc., Sydney, 10 mins.

Briggs, H. and Fisher, D. (2000) *Warning – caring is a health hazard: results of the 1999 national survey of carer health and wellbeing*, Carers Association of Australia, Canberra.

Cohen, L. and Manion, L. (1994) *Research methods in education*, 4th edition, Routledge, London.

Dansie, K. (2006) Trainee survey results, unpublished data.

Dowling, K. (2002) 'Africa's AIDS heroines'. *The Tablet*, 30 November, p. 7.

Fullan, M. (1993) *Changing Forces*, Routledge, London.

Hanks, P., McCleod, W. and Urdang, L. (eds) (1986) *Collins English Dictionary*, 2nd edition, Williams, Collins and Co., London.

HOME Hospice in South Africa 2006 documentary (2006) [DVD], HOME Hospice Inc. and Mannionfilms, Bundeena, 1 hr 50 mins.

HOME Hospice Inc. (1993–2009) Files, unpublished, Bundeena.

Kellehear, A. (1999) *Health promoting palliative care*, Oxford University Press, Melbourne.

Kellehear, A. (2005) *Compassionate cities. Public health and end-of-life care*, Routledge, London.

Manion, H.-A. (2006), *Free medicines*, HOME Hospice Inc., Sydney.

Manion, H.-A. and Manion, G. (1997a) *Coordinator's Manual*, HOME Hospice Inc., Sydney.

Manion, H.-A. and Manion, G. (1997b) *Notes for Carers*, HOME Hospice Inc., Sydney.

Manion, H.-A. and Manion, G. (1997c) *Preparing for the Final Farewell*, HOME Hospice Inc., Sydney.

Manion, H.-A. *et al.* (2009) "Where have all the elders gone: Transforming communities by reclaiming the wisdom of the past". 1st International conference on public health and palliative care, January 2009, Kerala, India.

Marcus, T. (2002) *Wo! Zaphela Izingane: It is Destroying the Children: Living and Dying with AIDS*, 2nd edition, November 2002, CINDI Network, Johannesburg, pp. 3, 32–35.

Martin, C. (2004) *Glow worms*, Kurisanani, Tzaneen RSA.

O'Leary, A. (2009) *Anti-retroviral program statistics*, [EMAIL] personal email from ART Coordinator Tzaneen RSA to H.-A. Manion [19 July 2009].

Rule, G. and Melele, R. (eds) (2004) "Theological and ethical issues in relation to HIV", speech by Munhedzi, T. at All-Africa conference: sister to sister: Southern Africa conference 20–25 April 2004, Bronkhorstspruit, South Africa, UISG Assemblies, Rome.

Sallnow, L., Kumar, S. and Kellehear, A. (eds) (2009) *1st International conference on public health and palliative care: January 2009: Kerala India*, University of Bath and Institute of Palliative Medicine India. Available at www. pubhealthpallcare.in (accessed 2 August 2009).

van Rijn, K. (2006) 'The AIDS debate: Thabo Mbeki and the South African response', *Social History of Medicine*, Vol. 19, No. 3, pp. 521–538.

Whitelaw, C. (2005) *Who was Granny Crabtree?* Whitelaw Publication, Batemans Bay.

Woods, P. (1997) *HOME Hospice: an interview with Christine Jones*, [Video recording] HOME Hospice Inc., and A. Manion Entertainment, Sydney, 15 mins.

Further reading

Africast (2004) *South Africans dying of hunger*, www.africast.com/health_article.php, (accessed 4 May 2004).

AIDS Foundation South Africa, 2002, ISISA Charities, www.isisa.co.za/isisa/aids/default.htm (accessed 11 November 2002).

Avert (n.d.) *AIDS orphans*, www.avert.org/aidsorphans.htm (accessed 30 March 2007).

Avert (n.d.) *HIV and AIDS in South Africa*, www.avert.org/aidssouthafrica.htm, (accessed 30 March 2007).

Caritas (2005) *Caritas Australia HIV/AIDS policy: Executive summary*, Caritas, Australia.

Carradine, B. (1999) GST speech: parliamentary debates (Hansard) senate. 14 May. Vol. 196, 39th Parliament, 1st session, 2nd period, p. 5117.

The Change is on – tools for pure living (2007) [DVD] Commissioned by the Diocese of Tzaneen, Metanoia Media Film, 49 mins.

Cheney, D. (2004) *Current and historical information about the bishops and Diocese of the Catholic-hierarchy*, Tzaneen Diocese, www.catholic-hierarchy.org/diocese/dtzan.html (accessed 5 June 2004).

Crabtree, B. and Miller, W. (1992) *Doing qualitative research*, SAGE, London.

Hausler, N. (2002) *African Women – HIV/AIDS*, Church Missionary Society of Australia, Victoria.

HOME Hospice in South Africa 2004 (2004) [DVD] HOME Hospice Inc., and Mannionfilms, Bundeena, 2 hrs 40 mins.

HOME Hospice in South Africa 2006: Documentary Short Presentation (2006) [DVD] HOME Hospice Inc. and Mannionfilms, Bundeena, 6 mins 52 secs.

Kraus, P., Andrews, S. and Tanchel, I. (2002) 'HIV Infection and its implications for palliative care in South Africa', *Progress in Palliative Care*, Vol. 10, No. 4, St Luke's Hospice, Kennilworth SA.

Lonely Planet (n.d.) *South Africa – History*, www. lonelyplanet.com//destinations/Africa/south_africa/history.htm (accessed 11 November 2003).

Marcus, T. (2004) *To live a decent life: Bridging the gaps: A study of SACBC programmes in support of orphans and vulnerable children in South Africa and Swaziland*, SACBC, Johannesburg.

Morgan, D., Mahe, C., Mayanja, B., Okongo, J. Martin, Lubega, R. and Whitworth, J.A.G. (2001) *HIV-1 infection in rural Africa: is there a difference in median time to AIDS and survival compared with that in industrial countries?* Lippincott Williams and Wilkins, London.

Morgan, D., Maude, G., Malamba, S.S., Okongo, M.J., Wagner, H.-U., Mulder, D.W. and Whitworth, J.A. (1997) 'HIV-1 disease progression and AIDS-defining disorders in rural Uganda', *The Lancet*, Vol. 350, 26 July 1997.

Rodrigues, M. (2003) "Where little children bury their parents", *The Catholic Weekly*, 16 March, p. 9.

Rule, G. and Melele, R. (eds) (2004) *All-Africa Conference: Sister to sister: Southern Africa conference 20th–25th April 2004*. Bronkhorstspruit, South Africa; UISG Assemblies, Rome.

Russel, M. and Schneider, H. (2000) *A rapid appraisal of community-based HIV/AIDS care and support programs in South Africa*, University of Witwatersrand, Johannesburg.

Silverman, D. (2000) 'Choosing a Methodology' in *Doing qualitative research: a practical handbook*, Sage, London, pp. 88–101.

Slattery, H. (2003) *HIV/AIDS: a call to action*, MSC Mission Office, Johannesburg.

Sowing in Tears – documenting the comprehensive response of the Diocese of Tzaneen,Limpopo Province, to the HIV/AIDS pandemic (2007) [DVD] Metanoia Media Productions, 60 mins.

Tindley, C. (1901) 'We shall overcome', [SHEET MUSIC] reproduction 1965 from Black Print Culture Collection, Philadelphia.

Tshabalala-Msimang, M. (2002) 'Rooting out stigma – combating discrimination', speech by Minister of Health, South Africa, at the 'People living with AIDS summit', 28 October, 2002, Midrand, RSA.

UNAIDS/World Health Organization (2003) *AIDS epidemic update*, December, UNAIDS/WHO, Geneva.

Uys, L. (2001) 'The practice of community caregivers in a home-based HIV/AIDS project in South Africa', *Journal of Clinical Nursing*, 11, pp. 99–108.

Uys, L. and Hensher, M. (2002) *The cost of home-based terminal care for people with AIDS in South Africa*, Vol. 92, No. 8, School of Nursing, University of Natal, Durban.

Vercoe, E. and Abramowski, K. (2004) *The grief book: strategies for young people*, Black Dog Books, Fitzroy Vic.

World Health Organization (2003) 'Global situation of the HIV/AIDS pandemic, end 2003', *Weekly epidemiological record*, No. 49, 78, WHO, Geneva, pp. 417–424.

World Health Organization et al. (1999) *AIDS home care handbook*. National AIDS Programme, TASO and country offices of UNICEF and WHO, Uganda.

World Health Organization/UNAIDS (2004) *Sub-Saharan Africa: AIDS epidemic update*, UNAIDS and WHO, Geneva.

World Health Organization/UNAIDS (2006) *Sub-Saharan Africa: AIDS epidemic update: Global summary of the AIDS Epidemic*, UNAIDS and WHO, pp. 19–25.

11 'Let's talk about dying'
Changing attitudes towards hospices and the end of life

Nigel Hartley

Introduction

This chapter explores the establishment and development of a death education project at St Christopher's Hospice, London. It provides some background information about St Christopher's Hospice and the current challenges that face both the organisation and end of life care in general. The responsibility that all hospices and end of life care providers have for promoting healthier attitudes towards their work, enabling society to shift its view of both death and dying is emphasised. The history of the St Christopher's Schools Project is presented together with a detailed project plan. Following this, material from a number of projects undertaken with different schools and colleges is discussed. Results from the project evaluation study are given before conclusions are drawn and new public education initiatives at St Christopher's Hospice are considered.

St Christopher's Hospice, London

St Christopher's Hospice, London, opened in 1967 and it was the inspiration of Cicely Saunders who worked in the new National Health Service of the 1940s and 1950s where 'dying was not part of the vision' (Monroe and Oliviere 2003). It aspired to be a place where dying could be accepted as a normal experience and well supported. In order to manage dying well, Saunders created the concept of 'total pain' (Clark 2002), which incorporates and addresses the physical, emotional, social and spiritual elements of those who are dying. The care and support of patients' families and carers was also central to her vision. In order to deliver the concept of total pain effectively, the development and comprehension of multi-professional working was key to Saunders's early work and has continued to remain at the heart of hospice care. A cohesive mix of care, education and research was also fundamental to the understanding and acceptance of end of life care from the start. The success of Saunders' early research into pain and symptom management was to change the face of medicine forever (Watson *et al.* 1993).

Although a uniquely individual response from Cicely Saunders to deficits she noticed in good end of life care, it was well planned:

St Christopher's will try to fill the gap that exists in both research and teaching concerning the care of patients dying of cancer, and those needing skilled relief in other long term illnesses and their relatives.

(Saunders 1967)

The St Christopher's building and inpatient wards were always central to Saunders' dream, but the endorsement of her much broader philosophy was captured with the first home care community nursing service which become operational in 1969 and also the first bereavement support service, with one of the first day care services following soon afterwards (Monroe *et al.* 2007).

The fact that Saunders' ideas and philosophy have spread so rapidly across the world has cemented the development of the modern hospice movement as one of the most successful humanitarian innovations of the twentieth century. Almost 45 years later, St Christopher's is one of the largest of around 300 hospices and specialist palliative care units in the UK, and as a result of its history holds a significant local, national and international reputation. Today, there are end of life care services in over 115 countries. As a local community provision, St Christopher's Hospice serves a population of 1.5 million people across South East London, taking in the London boroughs of Bromley, Southwark, Lewisham, Lambeth and Croydon. St Christopher's is a registered charity and costs over £14 million a year to run (as at 2010). It receives around a third of these costs from the National Health Service, with the rest of its income generated from other sources including legacies, voluntary donations and fundraising. The building includes four wards with 48 beds, and a day care and outpatient service known as the Anniversary Centre. On any one day the multi-professional staff team will provide medical, nursing, social, psychological and supportive care to over 800 patients and those who care for them within the places that they live, including care homes. St Christopher's is one of the largest suppliers of specialist palliative care education in the world. A purpose built education centre draws around 5000 students on-site every year with a further 2000 students being reached through outreach education programmes. The education centre runs approximately 70 training courses each year including an MSc in Palliative Care delivered jointly with King's College, London, and diplomas in both child and adult bereavement accredited by Middlesex University.

Despite the success of Cicely Saunders' vision with the development of hospices and end of life care across the world, there are still substantial challenges. An ageing population will mean that many more people will die in care homes and that people will live longer with multiple, chronic illnesses that will need to be supported. Families who live apart and are more widely scattered than in the past will struggle to care for their loved ones, putting more pressure on formal health and social care agencies. End of life care providers also have to face the challenge to find a way for currently excluded groups such as black and minority ethnic communities, those living in deprived areas, people with mental health problems and disabilities, refugees, asylum seekers, travellers, prisoners, the homeless, drug and alcohol mis-users, carers and those who do not have the 'correct disease' to access good care, when they need it, wherever they need it (Monroe et al. 2007).

Health promotion and death education

It is clear that from the outset the intention of the modern hospices was to provide and promote good quality end of life care (Clark 2002). However, provision and promotion have not always been easy bedfellows. Some years ago, it was stated that hospices provided 'deluxe dying for the privileged few' (Douglas 1992). This view of hospices has possibly developed from what might be seen as a dogged determination to furnish communities with an exemplar model for the provision of good quality end of life care. However, it could be argued that this kind of inward focus has led to hospices becoming increasingly isolated from mainstream health and social care providers, turning into 'silos' with little influence on, or partnership with, mainstream services. Institutions created solely to deal with the end of life might be accused of overlooking the importance of promoting and cultivating healthier attitudes towards death and dying within communities at large. One of the major failings of the modern hospice movement can be considered to be the minimal change in public attitudes towards death and dying. It is clear that many people are afraid of talking openly about the end of life, many people are afraid of contemplating the end of their own life and that of those they love, and many people are afraid of entering a hospice within their local community. However, those of us who work closely with people coming to the end of their lives know that their previous encounters with death and dying will contribute to their own experience as well as to the experience of those who are with them during the dying process. In 2008, the UK Department of Health published the first national End of Life Care Strategy. As part of calling for a joined-up, high quality end of life care service, it highlighted the consequences of a lack of public awareness and common debate about end of life issues and appealed for national engagement in order to radically change the way in which society views death, dying and bereavement.

Although a lack of openness about death and dying has been highlighted as a problem across modern society in general, there have been some exemplars of successful innovative development within the field of death education and public involvement. Allan Kellehear's books *Health Promoting Palliative Care* (1999) and *Compassionate Cities* (2005) present theories and examples of community development and strategies for implementing a public health programme around end of life care. Also, St Christopher's Hospice both pre-empted and responded to the UK Department of Health's national End of Life Care Strategy's call for action in a number of ways. A regular on-site professional concert series brings in members of the local community in order to enjoy high quality musical social events within the hospice building. This series enables people to come together with hospice users, staff and volunteers in order to enjoy being together and dispel myths about the work that St Christopher's does. Many people who attend the concerts talk of their preconceived perceptions and their denial of death and dying as being changed and challenged. The St Christopher's 'Community Choir' meets weekly and provides opportunities for members of the local community to sing and perform together with patients and their families. Also, regular public education events held at the hospice bring together specific community groups, such as faith leaders, those living with learning disabilities and others in order to learn about the work that is done and hopefully change attitudes towards the end of life. The St Christopher's Schools Project is another example of the responsibility the hospice acknowledges to work with the local community with the specific aim of providing opportunities to change the way in which people view death and the work of the organisation.

The St Christopher's School Project

Background

The St Christopher's Schools Project was set up in 2004/2005. It grew out an idea to bring together primary school children and dying people in order to provide an opportunity to examine if it was possible to unite two very different community groups so that they could learn from each other, changing perceptions of death and dying in a healthy and supportive way (Hartley 2007, 2011; Hartley and Kraus 2008; Hartley and Payne 2008). Although the project was driven by both St Christopher's vision and mission to change and promote positive attitudes towards the work that it does, it is important to highlight how the project also offered a series of 'quick wins' for schools and colleges and their own responsibility to the children and students that they educate. Loss and transition are part of the UK National School Curriculum (Department for Education 2005) and many schools find addressing these issues in a direct way difficult to manage. Other key requirements of schools to educate pupils about the impact of bereavement and separation and how to develop self-confidence and successfully deal with significant changes and challenges in life were also key drivers within the initial design of the St Christopher's Schools Project. It is sensible that the expertise and knowledge that hospices possess are used to support and address the aims of organisations that sit as part of the communities which they serve. It was therefore important from the outset that the project was driven by the needs of both the hospice and local schools in order to develop partnerships which would have the best chance of success for all involved.

Although it is familiar to come across schools and colleges who support the local hospice through fundraising activities, it is unlikely that any of these schools or colleges focus on educating pupils about the work that hospices do. From the outset, it was the aim of the St Christopher's Schools Project to enable children and hospice users to meet together directly in order to focus on changing attitudes in a straightforward way.

Guidance and information

The St Christopher's Schools Project is a structured, managed programme. Although flexibility has been important as it has developed and incorporated many more schools, colleges and other community groups, good planning and organisation has always been paramount. A practical guide was published in 2008 (Hartley and Kraus 2008) in order to share the project plan so that other organisations could see both the potential of hospices acting as centres for death education, and be offered guidance as how they could take the project, develop it to fit in with their own unique requirements and operate it successfully to fulfil organisational strategic objectives.

The project is usually set within a structure of four weekly meetings of two to three hours. However, there are a number of important issues to take into consideration as part of the pre-project planning and also important matters to address in between the more formal weekly meetings. The following gives a simple outline to the project in three parts.

Part one – identifying stakeholders and gaining commitment

The early planning stages of any project require commitment from all prospective participants. It is important to identify the key stakeholders at an early stage. At the outset of the schools project at St Christopher's Hospice, the following groups were identified as being paramount to the project's success:

- The hospice senior management team;
- The head teacher and class teacher of the school;
- Patients and their families;
- Children, students and their families;
- Hospice staff – nurses, bereavement and social workers, artists;
- Hospice volunteers.

It is clear that any of the above could have the potential to make or break the project, so working closely with them during the planning stages is essential.

Engaging school staff and parents

Meeting with the head teacher of the school helps to identify the most suitable age group of children who might benefit from the project. At St Christopher's we have found that in Primary Schools nine- and ten-year olds are the most suitable age group with 16- and 17-years olds being the most suitable age group in secondary schools. This is mainly because other age groups have important transitional events going on in their lives which require most of their attention and energy. However, over the years we have worked with many different age groups and experience has shown us that there is something different to be gained from doing the project with all age groups across the school education trajectory. Once the age group is agreed with the head teacher, it is important to engage the class teacher together with any classroom assistants who will be involved. These initial meetings are important in order to outline the aims and objectives and to allay any fears or difficulties individual staff may have as part of their own perceptions and experiences of both the hospice and the end of life. It is also important to identify any children who have been experienced bereavement in their families or other related life changing events. However, just because a child or student has been bereaved does not mean that they should not engage in the project. An informed decision regarding their involvement should be reached by including the child or student and their patients within the decision making process as well as including other key people. As the school are experienced in dealing with the children's parents and guardians, they should take on the task of informing them about the project. This is normally done by letter, but some schools offer a face-to-face meeting with parents in order to explain the importance of the project and their rationale for engaging with it. It has been rare that parents have refused their child's involvement with the project, mostly because they have been informed clearly and sensibly about the reasons behind the work, thus alleviating any fantasies or anxieties.

Engaging hospice staff and volunteers

Identifying key people within the hospice is vital. As well as involving staff who will be directly involved, such as day care nurses, artists, social workers and counsellors, it is important that staff across the whole organisation are informed about the project in order to gain their commitment and understanding. Some hospice staff will feel protective of the people they care for, sometimes to the extent that they may subconsciously take decisions on their behalf. It is important that they are introduced to the benefits that the project is able to bring to all involved. Volunteers can also be key in enabling the success of the project. An example from one hospice who took on the project highlighted the difficulties of engaging volunteers as they had been omitted from the planning stages of the project. Volunteers' commitment will be important as they sometimes have close relationships with patients and can influence the engagement and involvement of both patients and their families. Most members of a hospice senior management team should recognise the importance of hospices being able to lead on health promotion concerns. From a strategic perspective, changing attitudes towards the work that hospices do is cemented within the Department of Health's 2008 End of Life Care Strategy and hospices will recognise the significance of finding ways to address this. However, providing senior managers with a detailed, well thought out plan, as presented in the St Christopher's Schools Project guidance pack, should give them the confidence to engage with the possibility and potential that such a venture might bring, both to the hospice and its place within the local community. It will also help them to create a credible story to inform hospice trustees and any other crucial organisational supporters about the project.

Engaging patients and their families

Patients and their families, of course, make up one of the most important stakeholder groups. Their commitment and engagement is essential. Most hospice day care units have groups of patients who attend the hospice on a regular basis and will have been engaged with various group work initiatives as part of this. Our experience shows that many patients and their family members understand the need to change perceptions about the hospice and the work that it undertakes. Many patients will have gone through the uncomfortable process of being referred to the hospice day care unit. It is not uncommon that initial responses to such a referral will have been negative, as the differences between the fantasies about hospices and the realities of what they do and offer are sometimes severely mismatched. Many patients, once having taken the step to attend the hospice for the first time, have their fantasies challenged and transformed and are keen that others should hear about their experiences. It is not uncommon that patients feel motivated and inspired to work on changing the attitudes of children and others towards sickness and the end of life, stating regularly that discovering that they have something to teach whilst they are dying is both surprising and rewarding. However, it is important that patients who engage with the project do so willingly and with full knowledge of what is expected. One or two open meetings with patients and their families can help to encourage and guide their allegiance and also support them to define the project's aims and objectives themselves, so that the process can be as dynamic and as engaging as possible.

Part two – the project

It is important not to underestimate the significance of agreeing the responsibilities of all involved in the project during the initial planning meetings with key stakeholders. For example, just because the hospice is the prime initiator of the project does not mean that it should bear all of the financial costs. It might be that the school takes on the responsibility for providing transport for the children to and from the hospice, or agrees to provide essential materials in order that the project can fulfil the initial aims and objectives. Another example might be that the hospice agrees to provide refreshments during each of the project sessions. Although some of these issues might appear to be unimportant, they can have a direct bearing on people's experience of the project and its success.

The project is segregated into four weekly sessions. Beforehand, however, there are some important considerations to be taken into account. The school will have informed staff, children and parents about the project, as will the hospice have informed its staff, patients and their families. One important addition for the school is a lesson plan for the children prior to the project starting. This will include learning objectives for the children such as understanding the history and role of the hospice within the local community and beginning to appreciate the complexities and challenges of illness, death, dying and bereavement. These initial lessons are important in beginning to identify and secure both the understanding and resilience that the children will need during the project.

It will also be important to identify a common theme that the project will be built upon. At St Christopher's we have fostered a large team of artists to support the project, discovering that the arts can offer an indirect way of engaging with people of all ages about important issues in a manageable context where different groups of people can come together and focus on common issues without depending on the complexities of language (Hartley and Payne 2008).

The first project session

HOSPICE STAFF VISIT THE SCHOOL TO MEET THE CLASS GROUP AND TEACHERS

The aim of this visit is to show a DVD or photographic footage of the hospice so that the children have a concrete idea of the place they will be visiting later that day. An opportunity should be given for children to share any fears or anxieties. Time should be taken to help the children formulate the questions they wish to ask the patients that they will meet on the first visit. This visit normally lasts between 45 and 60 minutes and takes place in the morning.

CHILDREN AND THEIR TEACHERS VISIT THE HOSPICE FOR THE FIRST TIME

Children and their teachers visit the hospice and are given a tour of the building in small groups. Following the tour, there is an open session where they meet the group and their carers with whom they will work together over the coming weeks. This session is managed by one of the hospice staff, and it should be an opportunity for children and hospice users to meet and ask and answer any questions they may have for each other. Children have a way of asking straightforward questions in a direct manner. Our experience shows that if users are prepared for this, they will answer the questions asked just as directly and straightforwardly. Children and users may also talk about what they will do together over the coming weeks. They may agree on an arts topic, for example, or a common theme that will guide their work together. Following the formal question and answer session, refreshments are served in order to provide a more informal time to further get to know each other. Following this first meeting, it might be important that both the children and the users undertake some preparatory work in order to be ready for the next meeting. Also, school and hospice staff may need to spend some time collecting materials or props to help with the agreed project theme. This visit normally takes between 60 and 90 minutes.

The second and third project sessions

The second and third meetings take place on the same day a week and two weeks later. Children and users come together in order to focus on the project theme. These sessions normally last between two and three hours. Content and materials for the sessions will have been planned and collated during the interim period so that everything is ready in time for the meetings to happen. Although these sessions will be very practical, creating artwork or working towards a performance, time should be given and every effort made for conversations to take place and real learning to come about; during these sessions, powerful stories can be told and relationships formed.

The final session

The final session provides an opportunity for the culmination of the project. We have discovered that to treat this final meeting as a celebration gives a chance for all stakeholders to come together in order to focus on what has been achieved. It is important that any artwork is exhibited, or any performance worked on by children and users is presented. Children's parents and patients' family members and friends should be invited in order to witness what has been achieved. Experience has shown us that this can be an important event for the parents of the children. Many parents will have grown up within the community that the hospice serves, but may never have had the courage to come into the building due to their own fears and anxieties about the work that is undertaken there. We have learned that their attitudes and perceptions can also be changed, facilitated and led by their own children's experiences of having made significant relationships with people coming to the end of their lives. It is important that opportunities are given for anyone involved in the project to comment on what it has meant to them and on what they have achieved and learned. The final session ends with a party, enabling people to socialise and take time to say goodbye. The whole session lasts between 60 and 90 minutes.

Part three – evaluation and reflection

Post-project meetings are an essential way of reflecting on what has been achieved and also provide an opportunity to track project developments and pick out any key learning tips for the future. These meetings can take place in a number of formats such as school and hospice staff meeting either separately or together. On occasion, patients and carers have visited the school to talk to other school children about their experiences of having been involved. Artwork can also be taken to the school or other community venue in order to be exhibited or performed. We have found that exhibiting or performing the work in a number of key community venues can draw in other groups of people to further develop the potential and of changing attitudes and perceptions towards death and dying. At St Christopher's we always use a simple questionnaire which all participants are encouraged to complete at the end of the project. We have also undertaken more in depth evaluations, especially when we have managed to gain specific funding in order to undertake the project and need to feedback on experiences. At this stage, many schools will opt to include the project as part of their annual education programme and it is important to gain agreement of all involved about this possibility. It might be that the project occurs annually or bi-annually, depending on the other commitments of the various key stakeholders.

The St Christopher's Schools Project – some examples

At St Christopher's we have now undertaken the project almost 40 times with a range of different schools and colleges incorporating children and students of various age groups. Although a pre-arranged structure is always important and useful, each project needs the flexibility to take on its own unique process. It is important each time the project is undertaken that it is uniquely developed by the key personnel involved and is based around a specific theme, leading to possibilities for celebration, exhibition or performance. The celebration, exhibition and performance elements of the project provide a vital opportunity for what is achieved to be shared and therefore have an impact beyond those immediately involved. Two examples of different projects undertaken at St Christopher's Hospice follow.

Example one

The first school that we worked with as part of this project in 2005 was a one form entry primary institution in the London Borough of Lewisham. The school has 210 pupils on its school register, and like other schools in the area has a diverse range of pupils from different multi-cultural and special educational needs (SEN) backgrounds. The school sees itself as part of the local community with many of its staff and pupils regularly attending the adjoining church for worship, thus enhancing the sense of a 'family school'. As with many organisations within South East London, it will not be unusual to come across people who have had direct experience of the work of St Christopher's Hospice, together with a range of people who will have heard about its work but not had any reason to engage with it other than possibly a community fundraising event.

Since working with the school in 2005, the project has become an annual event as part of the Year Five educational programme. This means that to date five years' classes of children have engaged in the schools project.

Over the five years, the school has engaged with hospice users in many ways. However, the first time we did the schools project provides some useful examples of the types of questions the children ask patients when meeting them for the first time. Following a tour of the hospice during the first session of the project, a group of 30 ten-year olds and their teachers and classroom assistants met with around 15 patients both from the hospice day care unit and the hospice inpatient unit. We all sat in a circle and introduced ourselves. The patients told the children something about their illness and also about where they had been brought up and spent their early years at school. The children told the patients something about what they had learned about the hospice as well as something about the school they attended. It was interesting to learn that one of the patients had attended the school where the children were from when he was a child, and another patient's children had also attended the school some years earlier. Once the introductions were over, we asked both the children and the patients if they had any questions that they would like to ask each other. The questions from the children were direct and straightforward and included:

What is it like to have your breast cut off?
Why haven't you got any hair?
What happens to your body when you're dead?

Although many of the school and hospice staff appeared uncomfortable, it was interesting to note that the patients answered the questions in a frank and honest way. Many of us learned how easy it is for professionals to step in and stop things happening as we are concerned that it will be too uncomfortable or unbearable for those that we care for. However, this experience provided some invaluable learning. The patients that we care for are, for the most part, resilient human beings with a unique set of experiences that we can all learn from. During this exchange of questions and answers there can be no doubt that something beneficial and healthy was taking place. We learned that when managed and supported, difficult questions can be asked between two seemingly very different groups and lives can be changed. We were also given useful insights which were then taken forward and used in subsequent projects.

Example two

St Christopher's has worked with a number of secondary schools providing opportunities for older children to come together with hospice users. As the arts have been central to all of the projects at St Christopher's, students who are studying the performing arts have been keen to engage with us. Some of the projects have included patients and children writing, performing and recording songs together. Others have formed joint bands which have performed music that has been meaningful to people during their lives, whilst others have listened to patient stories and have transformed them into theatre performance pieces with the patients taking on the roles of both directors and actors in their own stories. The latter example of performing patients' stories as theatre has become the main driver for one local secondary school we have worked with regularly. When we first began working with teenagers, there was a reluctance from both patients and students to work together. This was based on a feeling that they had nothing to learn from each other. The first time we brought together a group of elderly patients coming to the end of their lives and a group of 16-year olds was an interesting experience. Their initial reluctance changed rapidly upon meeting each other, as they instinctively began to tell each other their stories. We learned that patients are keen to tell their stories to the teenagers, and are both surprised and humbled when their story becomes theatre, understood and performed with dignity and respect. Some stories are simple, whilst others are deeply moving and surprising. The following are just a few examples of stories shared as part of a recent schools project:

Story one

Hi, I'm Alison and I want to make the most out of what's left of my life. I enjoy spending time with my family; my children come and visit me a lot, which makes me happy. In my spare time I am busy making them special things ... I can't tell you what they are because it's a surprise.

Before I came here I enjoyed doing things a normal woman would do, like going out for drinks with my mates and driving my car. I would drive everywhere, discovering new places, I found it relaxing. I can't do that anymore. I can remember years ago I was in the car with my boyfriend at night, when it broke down in the middle of nowhere. I got out to find help but because it was so dark I couldn't see where I was going. I fell down a hole; I was stuck down there for ages until my boyfriend decided to rescue me. Unfortunately he was the one with the torch so he could actually see. But it's a good memory, I laugh whenever I think about it . . .

I suppose you'd like to know more about my illness, well I've got cancer, breast cancer. One day I woke up and just knew. . . . My breast had to be removed, but it wasn't over, it happened all over again. It also affected my neck, which I treated with radiotherapy, but that damaged my brain, which is why I have trouble walking.

My life has changed a lot, I wish my friends would treat me the same as they used to, I'm still the same person. I know they care but it's frustrating not to feel normal around the people I'm close to. When I was told I would be coming to St Christopher's my mind was filled with images of death and depression, hospice is not a nice word, so I expected to hate it. It's actually not that bad at all. Knowing that a lot of patients are suffering more than I am is a relief. I'm one of the lucky ones.

Story two

I'm Ronnie and I've been smoking about 52 years now, started quite young. I'd rather be outside in the sunshine having a cigarette now actually. No point of stopping now, you could say I'm beyond the point of return.

I remember waking up one morning and only just getting my socks on couldn't do anything else and then it was to the hospital. I couldn't tell my wife. I told the doctors 'no you tell my wife'. How could I tell the love of my life I had 6 months left to be with her?

Story three

My good people I'm Jeremiah. All you young people should treasure your lives. I am on a boat. We are back in the 1950s.On a boat called the Venezuela and we are sailing to England from Grenada. 18 days on that boat before arriving in England. I arrived in an England that is full of shouting and racists. It is blacks versus whites; bricks going through café windows and I am on the streets of Brixton. And the Brixton riots changed everything. Nowadays a black man can walk down the street with a white woman; no problem. I praise God I am still married to my wife. She is wonderful and has given me six beautiful children. My baby girl got married the other day. Fantastic wedding, food was brilliant – and cheap, we know the caterers so we got a good deal. We were begging people to take it home in containers at the end. Oh I've had a good life. I'm 74-years old and can still enjoy a brandy and coke.

Performances of patient stories have been taken across the world as a result of this project. Students from one school performed a series of patient stories at the European Congress of Palliative Care held in Vienna, Austria, in 2009. A similar performance has also been given within the Houses of Parliament in London. One of the most important things for people when they come to die is to tell their story to someone who is interested and who will give them their attention (Gunaratunam and Oliviere 2009). During the schools project many stories are shared, performed and witnessed. These stories illustrate for us the range and breadth of experiences that people carry with them towards the end of their life. The project gives the potential not only for patients' stories to be shared, but for the stories and the tellers both to have an impact on the young people's lives and for the storytellers themselves to leave something behind, changing young lives.

The St Christopher's Schools Project – evaluation

At the end of each project, a simple questionnaire is completed. It comprises a series of simple questions regarding the content of the project and includes space for free text asking for thoughts and feedback from the key stakeholders – patients, children and students, parents and staff. A content analysis has shown the emergence of key themes. These themes have helped us to ascertain and explicate important aims and objectives for the development of future projects. The four major themes are as follows:

Changing attitudes

When I first found out our community project was going to be at a hospice, I felt terrified and quite anxious about visiting St Christopher's. I didn't know much about hospices in general and I'd never heard of this one, so I had an image in my head of a stuffy hospital ward where people are sent to die. I was full of nervous energy when we first arrived, not knowing what to expect, but after ten minutes of being at St Christopher's, my view changed completely. Hospices do a difficult job and deal with tough issues, but St Christopher's is a wonderful place and seems to be doing a fantastic job of caring for the community, providing comfort to those who need it most. Someone working here hit the nail on the head when he told us on our first visit – "death isn't a disaster, it's the most natural thing in the world". This is so true, yet why do people still have an image of a hospice being a terrible place, somewhere to be feared and shunned? Something needs to be changed.

(17-year old)

...my grandmother died at the hospice and I wasn't allowed to go...I enjoyed seeing that it was OK really...

(Ten-year old)

Normalising death and dying

...at the start I felt a bit scared and shaky 'cos I thought it would smell and be full of sick people, but they were just normal...

(Nine-year old)

...we thought they'd all be miserable and depressed ... but it was just like being with your friends ... we laughed and cried and sometimes felt afraid, normal things...

(16-year old)

Patients as educators

...For the first time I feel my life has been worthwhile – really meant something. The students were amazed by my experiences and told me that they had learned something from me...

(Hospice patient)

...I always felt nervous talking to my children about what was happening to me – couldn't find the words and didn't want to upset them ... watching people talk to each other here gives me the confidence to talk to my own family...

(Hospice patient)

Creating and sustaining healthy relationships

...I'll always remember the patients, their stories and experiences. One guy in particular really made history being around London at that time ... he'll always be one of my heroes and I'll come back and visit him as long as he's alive...

(17-year old)

...I've lived in this area all of my life and have been too afraid to come into the building ... is it possible to volunteer some of my time to continue to help?...

(Parent of ten-year old))

Conclusion and future plans

Experience shows that public health campaigns can be an effective method of changing attitudes and public perceptions. During the AIDS crisis of the mid-to late 1980s in the UK, a powerful national advertising campaign about the dangers of unsafe sex (*Independent* 1993) significantly changed the potential development of the disease. Another current public health campaign in the UK has successfully given positive messages about healthy eating. The 'five a day' campaign, which fosters the benefits of eating five portions of fruit and vegetables every day gives a message which is now well known through a wide range of different UK communities and has been hailed as a marketing triumph (see www.dh.gov.uk). Although national programmes and marketing campaigns can be an important way of giving significant messages on a large scale, it is important that the activity of promoting healthier attitudes towards hospices, death and dying begins at a local level.

The St Christopher's Schools Project provides an effective model for hospices to begin to unravel the complexities of how society views them and the work that they do. The project has been mentioned as an exemplar in the Department of Health's End of Life Care Strategy (2008) and it has been developed effectively as part of many UK hospice programmes as well as having been delivered in other countries across Europe and the rest of the world. Recently, the partnership of a hospice and a local school in Australia won a major arts award for their own development of the St Christopher's School Project.

As a result of the success of the St Christopher's Schools Project, current initiatives include a programme which offers the possibility to roll out a similar scheme across local care homes. Three pilot projects have already shown the benefits of changing attitudes towards care homes and the elderly within their own communities. Funding has been secured from Arts Council, England, to further develop the project into the care homes of south London over the next two years. Plans include working with community groups other than schools, such as churches, pubs and further education colleges and universities.

Whilst remaining aware of the successes of the past 40 years, hospices have the responsibility to reflect on gaps in their services and to do all they can to create new relationships and partnerships which can furnish the communities that they serve with high quality, cost effective end of life care within what is becoming an increasingly complex and challenging world. The St Christopher's Schools Project not only shows what is possible, but also illustrates the potential that hospices have to continue to innovate and challenge and also to change the way that death and dying is both viewed and experienced.

References

Clark, D. (2002) *Cicely Saunders – Founder of the Hospice Movement Selected Letters 1959–1999*. Oxford, Oxford University Press.

Department for Education (2005) *The National Curriculum – handbook for secondary teachers in England*.

Department of Health (2008) *End of Life Care Strategy – Promoting high quality care for all adults at the end of life*.

Douglas, C. (1992) For all the Saints. *BMJ*, 304, 579.

Gunaratunam, Y. and Oliviere, D. (2009) *Narrative and Story-telling in Palliative Care*. Oxford, Oxford University Press.

Hartley, N. (2007) Resilience and Creativity. In *Resilience in Palliative Care – Achievement in Adversity*, Monroe, B. and Oliviere, D. (eds), Oxford, Oxford University Press.

Hartley, N. (2008) Managing Creative Arts and Artists in Healthcare Settings. In *The Creative Arts in Palliative Care*, Hartley, N. and Payne, M. (eds), London, Jessica Kingsley Publications.

Hartley, N. (2011) 'Letting it out of the cage: Death Education and Community Involvement. In *Governing Death and Loss – Empowerment, involvement and participation*, Conway, S. (ed.), Oxford, Oxford University Press.

Hartley, N. and Kraus, K. (2008) *The St Christopher's Schools Project – a guidance and information pack*. St Christopher's Hospice, London.

Hartley, N. and Payne, M. (2008) *The Creative Arts in Palliative Care*, London, Jessica Kingsley Publications.

Independent (1993) Political interference hindered war on AIDS. Available at www.independent.co.uk/news/uk/political-interference-hindered-war-on-aids-1494146.html (accessed 25 May 2011).

Kellehear, A. (1999) *Health Promoting Palliative Care*. Melbourne, Oxford University Press.

Kellehear, A. (2005) *Compassionate Cities*. New York, Routledge.

Monroe, B., Hansford, P., Payne, M. and Sykes, N. (2007) St Christopher's and the Future. In *Omega Journal of Death and Dying*, New York, Baywood Publishing Company Inc.

Monroe, B. and Oliviere, D. (2003) *Patient Participation in Palliative Care: A Voice for the Voiceless*. Oxford, Oxford University Press.

Saunders, C. (1967) In *Cicely Saunders – Founder of the Hospice Movement Selected Letters 1959–1999*, Clark, D. (2002), Oxford, Oxford University Press.

Watson, M.S., Lucas, C.F., Hoy, A.M. and Back, I.N. (1993) *The Oxford Handbook of Palliative Care*. Oxford, Oxford Handbooks Series, Oxford University Press.

12 Public health approaches to end of life in Ecuador

Avoiding suffering at the end of life – a health service issue?

Patricia Granja H.

Introduction and background

Over the past years, several strategies have been developed to allow greater access of the general population to health care in Latin America. This has included a change in the organization of services and the generation of new models of caring. The majority of these models, however, were designed by international agencies and have failed to reconcile the population character-istics that determine the organizational culture of health services and human resources, and the response of users and their families to them. Furthermore, end of life issues have not been recognized, or even discussed, in relation to these models. The process of dying has been assumed, paradoxically, to repre-sent a pathological process that requires institutionalization and professional management. Increasingly, the supply of health care services considered palliative in developed countries is poor in developing countries (Harding and Higginson 2005). There is limited access to what has been called "death with dignity" or "good death", defined by Marcos Gómez Sancho in 2005 as "the right that everyone has to terminate his life in a serene, peaceful process, without pain or other significant symptoms and surrounded by their loved ones".

A change of the paradigm in the Ecuadorian Constitution and a new model of health care are the starting points for palliative care development in Ecuador, with the understanding that care must go beyond health services. Basic chal-lenges include medical training, empowerment of the community by increasing their capacity to care for their own members, the generation of comprehensive public policies and the integration of palliative care into the Ecuadorian health system, taking into account the cultural and social dimensions of dying, death and bereavement.

Constitution and *Sumak Kawsay* (good living)

The latest Ecuadorian Constitution (2008) states that: "We, the sovereign nation of Ecuador, decide to build a new form of peaceful coexistence in diver-sity and harmony with nature, achieve the good life, the Sumak Kawsay." *Sumak*

Kawsay (the notion of good living) is a kichwa[1] phrase that aims to incorporate the Andean cosmovision as part of a new framework of political, legal and natural governance. Sumak Kawsay was also incorporated in the Bolivian Constitution (2007), recognizing for the very first time the multicultural nature of the nation. Sumak Kawsay proposes that nature is an important part of social being and recognizes the community as an inherent dimension of welfare. It follows, therefore, that they should influence care and welfare in the wider context. In the introduction of the Ecuadorian National Plan for Good Living, René Ramirez, the national secretary of SENPLADES,[2] defined good living as: "The satisfaction of needs, achieving quality of life and death with dignity, to love and be loved, a healthy flourishing of all people in peace and harmony with nature and the indefinite prolongation of human cultures (...)".

Over 70 percent of the Ecuadorian population is mestiza (mix of Indigenous and Caucasian) and kichwa is not the mother language for most Ecuadorians, which led to significant debate regarding the relevance and appropriateness of the Sumak Kawsay statement. Despite this, the concept of Sumak Kawsay had become one of the main goals of the current government and it is being incorporated into every plan that public institutions develop. The National Plan for Good Living 2009–2013 includes 12 objectives that aim to change the concepts of our economy and social system development. Despite this shifting emphasis, no notion of a good death or end of life issues have been mentioned in official documents.

A new model of health care

Ecuador is a small South American country, according to the last census around 14,000,000 people live in 283,000 square kilometers (INEC 2010). Ecuador is significantly different to other developing countries in terms of inequity, low health expenditure and barriers on access to health services. The Ecuadorian health system is fragmented and segmented: 30 percent of the population has no access to health services (see Figure 12.1). According to the National Accounts, total health expenditure is around 4–5 percent of the total Gross Domestic Product (GDP); 51.6 percent of this expenditure is provided from the public sector and the 48.4 percent from the private sector (Consejo Nacional de Salud 2007). Almost 88 per cent of the private expenditure comes from "out of pocket" spending; 66 percent of this related to medicine procurement.

It is in this context that a new model of health care, MAIS-FCI – "Modelo de Atención Integral en Salud Familiar Comunitario e Intercultural"[3] – has been proposed by the Ministry of Health, in an effort to satisfy the population needs and reinforce the principles and values of Renewed Primary Health Care through all life stages and across all levels of care.

The model recognizes access to health and health services as a human right: it states that health care must be free, universal, solidarity-based and will shorten the inequity gap.

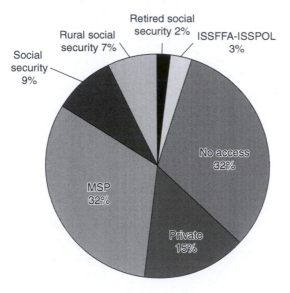

Figure 12.1 Health coverage in Ecuador (source: adapted from the Ministry of Health, Ecuador 2008).

Its principles, integrated in the holistic concept of Sumak Kawsay:

- include a deep respect of the culture of the population
- include a comprehensive approach of health and health determinants
- take into account various dimensions of care: individual, family and community.

The MAIS-FCI's functional unit is the EBAS (Equipos básicos de atención en salud, Basic health care team), which is responsible for the front line services with a strong home-visit component. Additionally, IESS, through a board resolution[4] (C.D. 308), incorporated in 2010 the principles of the Renewed Primary Health Care with the intention of transforming its services.

Even if end of life issues are not mentioned explicitly in the implementation draft of the MAIS-FCI, the principles and values of palliative care are totally consistent with it. Palliative care has been considered an important area of public health as it focuses on suffering, dignity, needs for care and quality of life of individuals and their families at the end of his life (Davies and Higginson 2004). Furthermore, the palliative care approach is the perfect example of a comprehensive, multidimensional strategy that demonstrates the feasibility of the new model of health care.

Could we avoid suffering?

Avoidability could be defined as the ability to prevent a disease (event) and/or its consequences (death, disability or loss of autonomy). Most importantly, it states the decision to deliver the best possible care to resolve individual or community health problems,[5] as warranty of the fundamental human right to health (Moreira 2009). This approach implies that most of the time a health problem could be prevented, solved or mitigated from different levels. The avoidability criteria have been proposed to set the priority health problems that must be solved by the Ministry of Health (Narváez and Moreira 2009).

In the framework of community participation, specific knowledge that describes the different conditions of life of communities and individuals living in them will allow the identification of avoidable health problems and therefore establish the criteria used to prioritize intervention (Tognoni *et al.* 2009). It is important to identify the avoidability of the event itself, its consequences or both. Besides, the approach of the problem should be considered, in some cases the health problem could be prevented mainly with a health care intervention, e.g. the polio vaccine. But, in most of cases, health problems need some intersectoral interventions that focus on improving health determinants.

This framework could be applied in the analysis of the main goal of palliative care: diminish suffering in the individual, familiar and communitarian dimensions in order to identify the interventions that should be planned based on knowledge of the particular context of each health system and the relationship between: supply (health service), demand (users) and needs (technical standards).

The ex-president and the "political opportunity"

For several years, palliative care advocates have been attempting to demonstrate the urgent need to discuss end of life issues in the Ecuadorian health system, albeit unsuccessfully. This changed in September 2010 when the Ministry of Health led a workshop that aimed to outline a National Cancer Policy with the main actors of the national health system. Tabáre Vasquez, former oncologist and Uruguay's ex-president, well known because of his fight against cancer, was the guest of honor. His presence captured the attention of the media and enhanced the event.

David Chiriboga Allnut, Minister of Health, who is a specialist in prevention and community medicine, opened the workshop with an insightful speech that addressed palliative care. The speech was prepared with a high level functionary who was aware of the role of palliative care and who also was involved in the selection of the speakers – which included two people from institutions that have been working in the field of palliative care for many years.

> I would like to share a few words regarding palliative care, which often is not taken into account in the health issues debate. There is a wrong

conception about palliative care when we limit it to the administration of drugs to relieve pain. This view is extremely restrictive, since palliative care is much more and also represents a significant element of the strategies for health promotion. Palliative care, means above all, to "give back" to the family the ability to take care of their loved one with cancer; it is to allow the terminally ill, to choose "where," "how" and "surrounded by whom" they want to die. It means that people have the right to die without pain and within a spiritual balance. In other words, there are entitled to have a "good death", which is nothing more than a more advanced dimension of good living.

(Extract from David Chiriboga Allnut, Minister of Health's speech, September 2010. Author's translation)

The political opportunity was clear; this was the perfect scenario in which it raise awareness of the need for palliative care, not just as part of a comprehensive Cancer Program, but as a need of the Health System nationally.

As a result of this, a subcommittee of palliative care was formed within CONASA (National Health Council), by a provision of the Minister, with the goal of drafting a proposal that would improve access to palliative care services. As a result of the subcommittee's work, in February 2011, the Minister of Health signed an accordance that recognizes the importance of palliative care and demands its integration across all levels of health.

Three core aspects, or areas of action, are developed in the accordance:

1   The organization and integration of palliative care services in all levels of care, in both public and private networking, under the framework of the new model of health care.
2   The access to pain relief drugs. Oral morphine is recognized for the first time as an essential drug.
3   The education and training of health workers on palliative care issues and the inclusion of palliative care in the curricula of health professions.

Although the accordance represents significant progress, there remains a significant void in the document: the lack of reference to community participation and the involvement of the terminally ill patients and their families.

In the next section an overview of the current state of each area of action will be presented.

Action area 1: organization and integration of palliative care services

The World Health Organization has recommended that palliative care services are included as part of national health policies for over a decade. To estimate the need for palliative care, mortality data were used, as shown in Table 12.1. However, this estimate omits a range of other chronic and life-threatening diseases. Additionally, it must be appreciated that there may be an underreporting

Table 12.1 Estimate of people requiring palliative care in Ecuador, 2008

Total deaths from cancer, cardio-cerebrovascular diseases and HIV/AIDS	Patients in need of palliative care	% of total population
11,548	9238 (80%)	0.1

Source: Adapted from: INEC, Anuario de estadísticas vitales, Nacimientos y defunciones, 2008.

of deaths. This may be due to the under diagnosis of malignancies due to lack of detection and recording, and issues relating to the registration of the primary cause of death.

The concentration of palliative care services for the total Ecuadorian population is one unit for every four million inhabitants. The majority of palliative care services are allocated in Quito and Guayaquil. Quito is the country's capital, located 2900 meters above sea level, with a population of 2,200,000. Palliative care services in this city are composed of:

- **ABEI Foundation** (Friends and benefactors of the incurables): Started in 1973 in Quito. At this moment, ABEI has a capacity of 65 beds for palliative care inpatients, chronic diseases patients and a long-term care facility, taking care of about 180 terminally ill patients each year. It also offers an outpatient care service.
- **FECUPAL** (Ecuadorian Foundation of Palliative Care): Created in 1997, its services include: outpatient care, in-home visits and follow-up calls. It also provides occupational therapy for most patients. This foundation takes care of about 250 patients per year. Even though services are limited to Quito, sometimes staff are able to attend people in near cities. FECUPAL is now building the first Ecuadorian Hospice, with 25 beds, which hopes to attend to 150 patients and families per year.
- **Jersey Foundation:** This multidisciplinary team provides outpatient care, home based care, a day hospice, follow-up calls and bereavement counselling, assisting 100 patients a year. It has been running since 2006. A parallel service works in the town of Santo Domingo, three hours away. It also provides educational palliative care programmes to health professionals and volunteers.
- **SOLCA-Quito** (League against cancer): This is the most important oncology hospital in the city, providing care for an average of 2200 new patients per year from all over the country. It offers outpatient care and interconsultation from other hospital services, registering a total of 1300 consults in a year, attended by three physicians. About four patients a month receive inpatient care, when this is essential.
- **Vozandes Hospital:** Offers outpatient care with an attendant average of 15 patients per year.

Guayaquil, located in the coastal region, is the most populated city in Ecuador, with 2,360,000 inhabitants. The main palliative care services are

SOLCA-Guayaquil, which offers outpatient and inpatient care, and a charity institution *La Casa del Hombre Doliente* (Grieving man's house), which cares for homeless people who are terminally ill.

All of these are non-profit private institutions and they depend on proceeds from charity, overseas funds, and out of pocket expenditure. An exception is SOLCA, in that it receives funds from the Ecuadorian government.

Services are isolated, no network exists currently and services are not integrated into the wider health system.

Main challenges for action area 1

- Shift the institution's paradigm from charity to a human rights approach.
- Assess the multicultural preferences and customs about dying, death, funerary rites and bereavement.
- Start a national network that integrates services across all level of health.
- Define the need for build new units that fit into the new "services typology" of the national health system.
- Define the core activities in the provision of palliative care for each level of care and its cost.

Action area 2: access to pain relief drugs

According to the International Narcotics Control Board (INCB), the morphine consumption in Ecuador during a year is 0.2 mg per capita, one of the lowest levels in Latin America. The global average consumption is 5.5 mg per capita, and the regional average is 1.7 mg. Cost is one of the main barriers to morphine access: a 10 mg morphine injection ampoule costs US$2.80, and a 20 mg injection costs US$3.20. A study conducted in Latin America showed that Ecuador has one of the highest average costs for morphine (Wenk *et al.* 2004). Assuming that an Ecuadorian patient needed the minimal dose of morphine (5 mg every four hours), that patient would have to pay approximately US$180 per month, equivalent to 68 percent of the Ecuadorian minimal wage (US$264) (Granja 2008). Other barriers include:

- Stock shortages.
- In order to prescribe potent opioids, physicians must be registered with the National Institute of Hygiene and pay a fee. The prescription expires after 72 hours.
- As in many other countries, myths regarding morphine use affect both prescription and consumption.
- The pharmaceutical industry's focus on the newer, more expensive opioids.

A significant achievement is that, as of February 2011, oral morphine features on the essential drugs list. Problems remain with availability. The National

Institute of Hygiene (INH) is responsible for warranty, access and availability and is required to present a technical proposal to resolve these issues in the coming months.

Main challenges for action area 2

- The use of the WHO's pain ladder as a tool for assessment and pain control.
- Lower morphine costs.
- Develop clinical practice guidelines for pain control and other symptoms.
- Improve bureaucratic process to prescribe opioids.

Action area 3: Education and training of health workers on palliative care issues

Across centuries, death has been conceptualized as an enemy to be feared and overcome; therefore, most training and practice for health professionals focuses on mechanisms that delay death. This is reflected in health care delivery and the health services organization model. In order to challenge and change this, end of life issues should be incorporated in the curricula of health professions at both undergraduate and graduate level. At the present time are some educative initiatives that include:

- A six-month course (diplomado) for nurses.
- An optional module of palliative care in a private medical school.
- A palliative care module for internal medicine residents.
- Short courses for both professionals and non-professionals on a yearly basis.

Currently, just a few health professionals have formal training in palliative care and the majority of those who do are concentrated in the capital. They do not represent sufficient human resources either to train further professionals or to effectively deliver care. Several strategies to train general practitioners and health workers over the country are currently being discussed. An effective referral system is essential and the use of new technologies such as e-learning and telemedicine should also be considered.

Main challenges for action area 3

- Define the general and specific competencies for palliative care in the health professions.
- Train EBAS (basic health care team) in the basic palliative care procedures.
- Develop cost-effective strategies to train people, discuss the roll of new technologies.

Key issues to be incorporate into the palliative care agenda

- To draft a conceptual model that includes the specific political, social and cultural determinants of health in the framework of the new health care model. This should also recognize dying as a life stage and community based palliative care as a feasible strategy to diminish suffering.
- To discuss the notion of "environments of care" as a social support model that involves community, health providers and decision makers and to propose global strategies that could be adapted locally in order to go from discourse into practice.
- To analyze how this approach could transform the medical training system from a "technology" paradigm to a "person focus" paradigm.

Conclusions and the way ahead

Enis Baris (1998) defined Health Policy and Systems Research (HPSR) as "the production of new knowledge and applications to improve how societies organize themselves to achieve health goals, including how they plan, manage and finance activities to improve health, as well as the roles, perspectives and interests of different actors in this effort".

The collection, analysis and discussion of relevant information in relation to palliative care from three approaches: supply (offer), demand and need in a health system, will allow us to understand the ideological factors and relationships that affect the delivery of care.[6] As palliative care services are proposed as a means of reducing the suffering of terminally ill patients, we must be aware of the concomitant risk of the medicalization of death (Clark 2002). The community should be involved from the outset. Numerous social, cultural and political aspects must be taken in account when drafting a prescriptive social support model with the aim of diminishing collective suffering. This must empower communities to care for their own members.

Palliative care should be understood on a community basis rather than be considered as just another health service. As Ira Byock said in 1997: "The nature of dying is not medical; it is experiential. Dying is fundamentally a personal experience, not a set of medical problems to be solved." Palliative care should be integrated in the new model of health care as well as in the design of a new model of medical training. These components are essential to go from the discourse into practice.

Notes

1 Spanish is Ecuador's official language. Nevertheless, the Ecuadorian Constitution recognizes kichwa and shuar as the official languages for intercultural relationship. Kichwa is an Andean language spoken by indigenous people, mostly in Ecuador, Bolivia and Peru.
2 SENPLADES (Secretaria nacional de planificación y desarrollo) is the Ecuadorian National Secretariat of planning and development.

3 A comprehensive, familiar and intercultural model of health care.
4 The IESS (Instituto Ecuatoriano de Seguridad Social), part of the national system, has financial and legal independence.
5 Understood as a given situation that limits either the individual or community autonomy and involves suffering.
6 Understanding ideology as "the system of beliefs that legitimate domination and resistance, marking the life of the social institutions".

References

Baris, E. (1998) *Defining and delimiting the boundaries of the Alliance for Health Systems and Policy Research*. Geneva, Background document, Alliance for Health Policy and Systems Research.

Byock, I. (1997) *Dying Well: The Prospect for Growth at the End of Life*. New York: Riverhead Books.

Clark, D. (2002) Between hope and acceptance: the medicalization of dying. *BMJ*, 324: 905–907.

Consejo Nacional de Salud (2007) *Política Nacional de Medicamentos*. CONASA 2007; 12.

Davies, E. and Higginson, I. (2004) *Hechos Sólidos en cuidados paliativos en Europa*. OMS.

Granja, P. (2008) *Análisis de la disponibilidad de opioides en Ecuador*. Available at www.saluddealtura.com/informacion-profesionales-salud/actualidad-medica/cuidados-paliativos-analgesicos/.

Harding, R. and Higginson, I. (2005) Palliative care in sub-Saharan Africa. *Lancet*, 365: 1971–1977.

INEC (2010) Preliminary data. Available at www.inec.gob.ec/preliminares/somos.html (accessed on 12 March 2011).

Moreira, J. (2009) *Ficha técnica de evitabilidad*. Bol. Epid. (Ecu) 2009; 6(57).

Narváez, A. and Moreira, J. (2009) *Priorización de enfermedades*. Bol. Epid. (Ecu) 2009; 6(7–27).

Tognoni, G., Prandi, R. and Marquez, M. (2009) Methods and actors of EPICOM. *Italian Journal of Tropical Medicine*, 13: 11–16.

Wenk, R., Bertolino, M. and De Lima, L. (2004) Analgésicos opioides en Latinoamérica: la barrera de accesibilidad supera la de disponibilidad. *Medicina Paliativa*, Vol. 11, No. 3: 148–151.

Appendix 1

Palliative care policy for Kerala

The Government of Kerala

1 Pre-amble

1.1 *The suffering in incurable and debilitating diseases:*

a   Life with an incurable and debilitating disease is often associated with a lot of suffering. Pain, many other symptoms like breathlessness, nausea and vomiting, paralysis of limbs, fungating ulcers etc can make life unbearable not only for that person, but also for the family. Such suffering exists in incurable cancer, HIV/AIDS, many neurological, pulmonary, cardiovascular, peripheral vascular and end-stage renal diseases, incapacitating mental illnesses and in problems of old age.

b   In addition to physical problems, they usually suffer from social, emotional, financial and spiritual issues caused by the illness. Many have clinical states of anxiety or depression. On the social domain, when wage-earners get the disease, in the absence of any social security system, families often get financially ruined. Cost of treatment adds to the problem. It may lead to their children dropping out of school; families losing their homes, and often going into debt.

1.2 The relevance of palliative care

a   Modern Principles of palliative care can take care of the suffering in patients with incurable diseases, considerably diminishing the anguish for the patient and the family. Palliative care is aimed at improving quality of life, by employing what is called "active total care", treating pain and other symptoms, at the same time offering social, emotional and spiritual support.

b   The World Health Organization in 2002 defined palliative care as "an approach that improves the quality of life of patients and their families facing the problems associated with life-threatening illness, through the prevention and relief of suffering by means of early identification and impeccable assessment and treatment of pain and other problems, physical, psychosocial and spiritual.

Palliative care

- Provides relief from pain and other distressing symptoms
- Affirms life and regards dying as a normal process
- Intends neither to hasten or postpone death
- Integrates the psychological and spiritual aspects of patient care
- Offers a support system to help patients live as actively as possible until death
- Offers a support system to help the family cope during the patient's illness and in their own bereavement
- Uses a team approach to address the needs of patients and their families, including bereavement counselling, if indicated
- Will enhance quality of life, and may also positively influence the course of illness
- Is applicable early in the course of illness, in conjunction with other therapies that are intended to prolong life, such as chemotherapy or radiation therapy, and includes those investigations needed to better understand and manage distressing clinical complications.

c   In a study done in Malappuram District of Kerala (it was found that around 40 per cent of those people who are dying would have benefited from applying the principles of palliative care in their management. In Kerala, with a population of 32 million and a crude death rate of 6.3 (Reference: Census 2001) around 80,000 dying patients and their families would be benefited each year. To this if we add the number of people living for years with chronic conditions the total number will be much more.

d   To ensure that palliative care is available and accessible to the majority of the needy, a major thrust should be on a primary health care approach. World Health Organisation observes that "The fundamental responsibility of health profession to ease the suffering of patients can not be fulfilled unless palliative care has priority status with in public health and disease control programme; it is not an optional extra. In countries with limited resources, it is not logical to provide extremely expensive therapies that may benefit only a few patients, while the majority of patients presenting with advance disease and urgently in need of symptom control must suffer with out relief" (National Cancer Control Programmes, Policies and Managerial Guidelines. WHO, Geneva 2002).

e   Even when the disease is amenable to curative treatment, especially if the treatment is a long-drawn out process like in cancer, all principles of palliative care need to be applied from the time of diagnosis. This is commonly called supportive care and needs to be incorporated into the disease-specific treatment program.

f   Palliative care is a well-established branch of health care in most developed countries. The state, under Article 21 of the constitution of India, is duty-bound to ensure the fundamental right to live with dignity. This policy is aimed at ensuring that palliative care services are established and integrated into routine health care in the state.

1.3 *Present palliative care scene in Kerala*

a   At present there are around 100 palliative care units in Kerala. Majority of them are:

- organised and supported by Community Based Organisations (CBO) and the rest are based in government and private hospitals
- supported by local communities
- self-sustainable in terms of manpower, money and other amenities
- dependent on trained volunteers for organising the services and psychosocial support
- supported by Local Self Governments Institutions (LSGI) and are
- able to provide home visits, outpatient service and free drugs for the poor.

In some districts however, palliative care services are rudimentary.

b   Currently palliative care training programmes for professionals are run by Institute of Palliative Medicine, Kozhikode and Regional Cancer Centre, Thiruvananthapuram. Calicut Medical College has been offering regular placement in palliative care for house officers as part of training.

c   There are around 4000 trained volunteers in palliative care in Kerala at the moment. About 25 doctors, 15 staff nurses and 50 trained nurses are working full time in palliative care in the state. I addition to this there are many health care professionals who contribute part of their time for palliative care.

2 Aims and objectives

2.1 *Aim: to provide palliative care to as many of the needy in Kerala as possible*

2.2 *Objectives*

2.2.1 *Short-term objectives for the first two years*

a **2.2.a.1.** To train at least 300 volunteers in palliative care in each district to facilitate the development and involvement of CBOs with emphasis on districts where there are no palliative care facilities.

2.2.a.2. To conduct sensitisation programmes in pain relief and palliative care for 25 per cent of all doctors, nurses and other health/social welfare workers in the state

2.2.a.3. At least 150 doctors and 150 nurses in the state to successfully complete Foundation Course in Palliative Care. (Ten days 'hands on' training in Palliative Care with three days/20 hours of interactive theory sessions)

2.2.a.4. At least 50 more doctors and 50 more nurses in the state to successfully complete six weeks training in palliative care (Basic Certificate Course in Palliative Care). In addition to this availability of essential drugs including oral morphine and protected time for trained professionals and provision for inpatient beds where appropriate to be ensured in government hospitals having doctors and nurses successfully completed six weeks courses.

2.2.a.5. To develop more than 100 new community based palliative care programmes with home care services in the state with active participation of CBOs, LSGIs and local government and other health care institutions.

2.2.a.6. To develop common bodies/platforms in at least 25 per cent of the LSGIs to coordinate the activities of CBOs, LSGIs and local health care programmes in the field of palliative care.

2.2.a.7. To establish a palliative care service, with availability of essential drugs including oral morphine and with at least one trained doctor and trained nurse, in all government medical college hospitals in the state and in district hospitals in districts without medical college.

2.2.a.8. To integrate the provision for palliative care into the house visit and field level activities of the field workers (Junior Health Inspector and Junior Public Health Nurse) and their supervisors.

2.2.a.9. To make essential medicines for palliative care available to patients covered by palliative care services through palliative care units/ Primary Health Centres/other government hospitals.

2.2.a.10. To develop at least four more training centres in the state for advanced training in palliative medicine and nursing.

2.2.a.11. To develop and incorporate palliative care modules in medical, dental, nursing, pharmacy and paramedical courses.

2.2.a.12. To introduce palliative care in to the training programmes for elected members to LSGIs and concerned officials.

b   Long term objectives (five–ten years)

2.2.b.1. To ensure the presence of at least 1000 active volunteers trained in palliative care in each district at any time.

2.2.b.2. To make community based palliative care programmes with home care services available to most of the needy in the state with active participation of CBOs, LSGIs and local health care programmes

2.2.b.3. To develop common bodies/platforms in most of the LSGIs to coordinate the activities in the field of palliative care of CBOs, LSGIs and local health care programmes.

2.2.b.4. To ensure the presence of the minimum necessary trained professionals in palliative care in each district. This will mean all the doctors, nurses and other health/social welfare workers sensitised; Minimum of 75 doctors and 75 nurses to complete foundation course; Minimum of 25 doctors and 25 nurses to complete six week course in palliative care. There should be a mechanism to utilize the services of trained professionals in the delivery of services.

2.2.b.5. To empower the LSGIs in the state to develop programmes for training volunteers in palliative care and facilitating the development and involvement of CBOs.

2.2.b.6. To develop a system of monitoring the palliative care service in the state to facilitate quality assurance. A guideline for quality control to be developed at state level with a monitoring/implementing mechanism at the district level.

2.2.b.7. To develop a system to document and compile data on the palliative care related activities and patient population at district and state level.

2.2.b.8. To continue training and facilitation to empower community to share the care and support of people needing palliative care by organising human and financial resources available locally

2.2.b.9. To develop post graduate courses in palliative care in Medical and Nursing Colleges in the state

2.2.b.10. To establish Palliative care as part of basic health care available at the community level

3 Development of services

3.1 *Guiding principles*

a   Home based care should be the cornerstone of palliative care in the state. The role of family in the care of chronically ill patients should be recognised. They should be socially supported and empowered to cope with the situation. The patient and the family should be the focal points of the palliative care programmes.

b   Palliative care should be part of general health care system of the Government machinery.

c   The three tier governance system in Kerala in which health care institutions up to the district level are transferred to the LSGIs, gives good opportunity for the LSGIs to facilitate the development of pain and palliative care services through the existing network of institutions in co-ordination with CBOs and community in general.

d   Field level health workers and their supervisors should be able to incorporate the principles of palliative care into their routine activity at the household level. For this purpose the existing manpower and institutions in health need to be oriented and equipped adequately.

e   The Government machinery will make use of the experience that CBOs/non-governmental organisations (NGOs) have acquired in training and delivery of palliative care in the state and will work with them.

3.2 Involvement by different sectors

a   **Government Sector:** There should be adequate facilities in govt. hospitals and other health institutions for providing palliative care services at the institutional level and field level. They are expected to work closely with the CBOs and NGOs under the overall co-ordination of the LSGIs.

3.2.a.1. Field level and Sub Centre level activity: Male and Female Multi purpose health workers, who are expected to provide the components of comprehensive primary health care services at the household level through the sub centres and at the PHCs, can be provided with the necessary orientation cum skill development training to play a major role along with the CBO volunteers and family members in providing home based care. CBOs and LSGIs should be encouraged to participate in palliative care delivery at this level.

3.2.a.2. Primary Health Centres and Community Health Centres: The Primary Health Centres (PHCs) and Community Health Centres (CHCs) in the rural areas should be empowered to provide the necessary institutional level palliative care. Through the necessary training programmes and by filling the critical gaps in availability of drugs and other components of service provision, these institutions are to be equipped for the above purpose. The medical officer of the PHC/CHC will have a crucial role along with the CBOs and the LSGIs in developing a common platform for the co-ordination.

3.2.a.3. Taluk Head Quarters hospitals: Where ever the existing palliative care services are located at far away centres, efforts should be made to provide full fledged palliative care services in Taluk hospitals. Efforts should also be made for the integration of the pain and palliative care concepts and skills into the existing specialty services of the Govt. Hospitals

3.2.a.4. District Hospitals & Medical Colleges: Each district must have a tertiary level pain and palliative care service with a trained doctor and staff nurse, housed either in a medical college Hospital or a District Hospital. They should have specialist and inpatient palliative care services and ideally, facilities for training too.

3.2.a.5. Creation of training centres: More training centres need to be developed in the state. In addition to training centres which may evolve in the NGO/CBO sector, efforts should be made to start more training centres in government sector.

b **Community Based Organisations (CBOs):** Issues associated with patients needing palliative care are as much social as emotional or physical. The society can pool its resources through CBOs to address many of these issues. As shown by experience in some Northern districts of Kerala, there is tremendous improvement is palliative coverage where CBOs are active. So participation of CBOs in palliative care should be encouraged.

3.2.b.1. Proposed minimum criteria for involving CBOs in palliative care.

a   They should be local organisations having clearly stated interest in the care of patients with needing palliative care in their area.
b   The organisation should take the lead role in providing home care services to the bedridden patients.
c   Should not charge patients or family for their services.
d   The persons involved in the care of patients needing palliative care – volunteers, nurses, doctors and other health care workers – should have basic training in palliative care.

3.2.b.2. Responsibilities of CBOs

a   Identify patients needing palliative care in the area with the help of Local Self Governments (LSGI).
b   Assess the needs of each patient and provide care accordingly.
c   Provide home care service for needy patients.
d   Empower the patients and their families; provide social support and rehabilitation where ever necessary.
e   Conduct awareness programmes in palliative care for the community and provide training for volunteers and health care workers.
f   Work together with Local Self Governments and the Government/ Non Government Health Institutions in the area for improving the care received by the patients.

3.2.b.3. Identification of CBOs: With the help of palliative care programmes in the neighbourhood, the LSGIs can identify and support CBOs.

3.2.b.4. Support for CBOs

a   Local Self Governments can take initiative to form a common platform for CBOs, Governmental and Non Governmental Health Institutions for organising support to the patients and family.

b   Local Self Governments should take steps to provide medicines and other accessories to the poor patients with chronic diseases identified by the CBOs, with the help of Government health care system.

c   **Private Sector:** Private sector plays a major role in the health care scenario in Kerala. Many private hospitals in Kerala are providing palliative care to needy patients free of cost. Palliative care initiatives by private hospitals should also conform to the quality control and training criteria set by the palliative care policy.

4 Capacity building

In Kerala at any time there may be a minimum of one lakh people needing palliative care. So each Panchayat will be having approximately 100 patients at any given time. To give adequate care to these patients there should be at least one doctor and two nurses trained in palliative care in every Panchayath to work along with CBOs and other health care institutions. Also there should be enough trained volunteers for effectively organising and running the programme at local level.

a   **Capacity building in government sector:** Considering the higher prevalence of the Non Communicable Diseases including cancers in Kerala, the significant number of people with HIV/AIDS and due to the increase in the percentage of the elderly population and the associated conditions requiring the palliative care services, it is essential that the health staff including the doctors are equipped with adequate technical and humanitarian skills for dealing the pain and palliative care services in a systematic manner.
4.1.a.1. Palliative care sessions will be built into existing educational programs (some of them are given in appendix V)
4.1.a.2. Deputation of staff will be given for the following training programs:
4.1.a.2.1. One to two day sensitisation programs in palliative care arranged for the purpose in collaboration with existing training programs in the field.
4.1.a.2.2. 10 day foundation course on pain relief for doctors and nurses. This course will authorise the doctors to man Recognised Medical Institutions (RMIs) which can store and dispense oral morphine and can provide basic pain relief to the needy.
4.1.a.2.3. Six weeks' certificate course for doctors and nurses in approved centres.
4.1.a.2.4. Other training programs yet to be developed for other categories of staff including pharmacists, public health nurses, health inspectors etc.

b   **Capacity building at CBO/NGO level:** There are many NGOs and CBOs actively involved in palliative care training programmes for doctors, nurses and volunteers. Along with supporting these initiatives these training programmes should be validated and guidelines given. The experience the NGOs and CBOs have in training can be used to formulate and initiate palliative care training programmes in government sector. There should be efforts from governments, CBOs and NGOs to recruit and train more volunteers at local level.

5 Availability of medicines and other equipments

5.1 A palliative care programme cannot exist unless it is based on a rational drug policy. Persons with incurable and other chronic illnesses need medicines for prolonged periods, which they may not be able to afford. In many areas CBOs and NGOs are now providing medicines and other equipments, which is not enough to cover the enormous needs in the state.

5.2 Medicines commonly needed for palliative care should be included in the essential drug list of the government hospitals. (Appendix II: List of medicines to be added to the present 'Essential Drug List') Also LSGIs should have provisions to purchase and distribute medicines and other equipments based on the need in their area with the help of health care institutions and CBOs.

5.3 There should be clear and adequate guidelines for procuring, storing and dispensing medicines needing special licenses like morphine. (Appendix III: Guidelines on training)

6 Role of other systems of medicine

6.1 Currently palliative care services are developing more as part of Modern Medicine. The possibility of having similar programmes in other recognised systems of medicine should be explored.

7 Research

7.1 There should be provisions for locally relevant audit and research at various levels for improving the programmes and for sharing the experiences.

8 Budget allocation

8.1 There should be separate provision for budget allocation for palliative care services under

    a   Directorate of Health Service
    b   Directorate of Medical Education
    c   Local Self Government Institutions
    d   National Health Programmes
    e   Employees State Insurance Scheme

8.2 There should be provisions for deputation of government doctors and nurses to palliative care services for supporting clinical work and training programmes.

9 Palliative care policy and other health programmes

9.1 Palliative care can be a component of many health programmes like National Cancer Control Programmes, National AIDS control Programme, National Noncommunicable Disease Control Programme, National Rural Health Mission etc. The state palliative care policy is also in line with these related health care programmes.

10 Evaluation and monitoring

10.1 It is necessary to evaluate the progress of the program at the end of one year, so as to analyse the strengths and weaknesses of the system and to formulate strategy for the long term policy. An advisory panel of palliative care workers will be formed comprising of representatives of the concerned government departments along with palliative care workers. The annual review will be followed by a revision of the short-term strategy for the second year, as well as the formulation of a long-term strategy.

Appendix 2

Charter for the normalisation of dying, death and loss [draft statement]

International Work Group on Death, Dying and Bereavement

The authors of this document are members of one group participating at the 2004 Tucson meeting of the International Work Group (IWG) on Death, Dying and Bereavement. These members are: Elizabeth Clark, John Dawes, Lynne Ann DeSpelder, John Ellershaw, Jack Gordon, Glennys Howarth, Allan Kellehear, Barbara Monroe, Patrice O'Connor, Lu Redmond, Marilyn Relf, Louise Rowling, Phyllis Silverman (Chair), and Diana Wilkie.

A group of members of The IWG on Death, Dying and Bereavement prepared a draft statement advocating the promotion of a public health perspective in all direct service approaches to end of life care. This statement, which we have called a Charter, is a draft of work in progress. Readers are invited to contribute their criticism, reflections and/or additions to this document by sending their thoughts to the authors via Phyllis Silverman at the contact address provided. All such contributions will be debated and discussed at the next meeting of the IWG held in Hong Kong in late 2005.

Introduction

The idea of developing this 'Charter' grew out of a discussion at the 2004 IWG for Death, Dying and Bereavement meeting in Tucson, Arizona, USA. It was stimulated by an article in The New Yorker magazine by Jerome Groopman on January 26, 2004 entitled 'The Grief Industry'. The article raised many questions about the nature of the care offered for bereaved people. The group saw this as a challenge to the medicalization of grief and its consequences for how death is viewed in Western society. We took this a step farther to consider how dying is dealt with as well. This is a working document. It is published at this time to invite responses from readers of this journal. In the medical model, the focus is on the 'body' and on medical care. This focus can be an isolating experience for the dying person and the people caring for him or her. This shortcoming results from a lack of community involvement and consideration of death as a fact of life. We began to seek ways of bringing the wider social context into the picture of death, dying, loss and care. As our discussion continued in this direction, we found ourselves moving toward a public health approach focusing on the promotion of competence and on the universality of needs arising from the inevitability of death and loss. Drawing on the experience of those of our members who have backgrounds in Public Health and who are applying this model in their current work, we developed the idea of a Charter. Similar to World Health Organization charters, this charter is a mission statement that describes ideal professional actions and values to strive for so that these eventually become benchmarks of everyday practice.

Purpose of the Charter

In relation to dying, death and loss, public health has frequently assumed the old medical view of death as failure, rather than recognizing and accepting it as a fact of life. On the other hand, service providers involved in end of life care have commonly overlooked the need to strengthen and build on the social potential of the communities they seek to support. The shortcomings of these two individual approaches to dying, death and loss commonly result in scepticism and criticism of both public health and end of life care services and initiatives. This Charter is a response to these problems. It brings the strengths and distinctive expertise of the two fields together in community building and death, dying and loss, respectively. This combined approach can facilitate knowledge transfer across each field that will enhance our joint goal of developing a seamless health care response toward the human experiences of death, dying and loss. This renewed approach includes the recognition of the importance of both community development and care of the individual (see Figure A2.1). The purpose of the Charter is to highlight the need for permeability between direct service provision and the growing community need for normalisation of dying, death and loss. Towards this aim, the Charter outlines the Essential Elements, Action Principles, Action Areas and Strategies for a comprehensive Public Health approach within the field(s) of End of Life Care. This charter builds on the earlier vision of the World Health Organization Ottawa Charter for Health Promotion (1986).

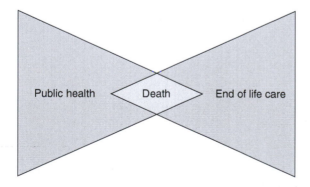

Figure A2.1 The challenge.

Definitions of the key terms

By Public Health, we mean the pursuit of the goals of prevention, early intervention and harm minimisation within all end of life care policy and practice initiatives that build community capacity through community development, education, participatory health care approaches, legislative and policy change. By End of Life Care, we mean all the support and services for people (i.e. direct services and informal care by families and communities) affected by the human experiences of dying, death, loss and the burden of care and their related experiences, consequences and changes.

Examples of services may include (but are not confined to):

- Care of the elderly
- Hospice and palliative care
- Bereavement care
- Services for chronic illness
- Accident and emergency care.

Essential elements of a public health approach toward end of life care

- Recognition of the inevitability of death and the universality of loss
- Cultural sensitivity and adaptability
- Culture/settings approach
- Social justice by promoting equal access for all
- Population health approach
- Sustainability.

Action principles

- Advocate [A]
- Enable [E]
- Mediate [M].

Action areas

1 Build policy
2 Create supportive environments
3 Facilitate community action
4 Develop personal skills
5 Re-orient health services.

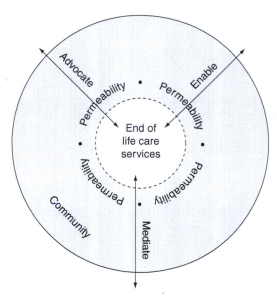

Figure A2.2 Action principles.

Strategies

Letters and numbers following each strategy denote their relationship to action principles and action areas:

1 Advocacy of the 'normal' (and recognition that the normal can be painful) [A]
2 Imaginative involvement and partnerships with community bodies [2/3]
3 Ensure access and choice from the community's perspectives [2/3]
4 Actively promote community development [3]
5 Mandate the participation of people using services [1]
6 Political lobbying by services and lead organisations within the community [1]
7 Target legislative changes [1]
8 Promote intersectoral collaboration [1/5]
9 Develop media partnerships [2]
10 Adopt a social marketing approach [3/4]
11 Provide public health resources for end of life care [5]
12 Develop a media communication role for lead organisations [1/2]
13 Promote education and supervision (interdisciplinary, cognitive and affective, critical and reflective) [4/5]
14 Promote communication between diverse health organisations about their common needs in relation to death and loss especially in respect of their common, diverse or absent languages [4/5]

15 Combat professional paternalism [4/5]
16 Ensure a collaborative approach to needs, definitions and outcomes [M]
17 Promote 'action' and 'practice' research priorities [E].

Call for international comment

The IWG on Death, Dying and Bereavement calls on all practitioners, academics and policy-makers to advocate the promotion of public health in all direct service approaches to end of life care, as directed toward our joint experiences in death, dying and loss. We affirm that the above Charter is a draft work in progress and invite all readers to contribute their criticism, reflections and/or additions to this Charter by sending their comments to the authors via Phyllis Silverman. All such contributions will be debated and discussed at the next meeting of the International Work Group held in Hong Kong in late 2005.

Appendix 3
Practice guidelines for palliative care

Allan Kellehear, Gail Bateman and Bruce Rumbold

1   i   Extend the activities or complement existing support groups with additional adult learning groups:

    a   Should be small groups (5–7 people maximum)
    b   Should have weekly reading material
    c   Readings should cover one's own health care and life changes but be flexible to the needs of the group
    d   There should be some component of death education
    e   Learning groups should run for a limited number of weeks (eg, 6–8 weeks)
    f   Ideally learning groups should be for patients only but if this is not possible or desirable at all times then a specific number of sessions should be put aside for carers only and patients only. These can be some part of any program where joint sessions are the main feature.

Two small group programs a year recommended

And/or

    ii   Offer opportunities for one-on-one patient information sessions with a health educator about life-changes, health maintenance and death education needs.

2   Demonstrated evidence of Death Education for:

    a   Patients
    b   Staff (including Volunteers)
    c   Caregivers
    d   Community (talks, publications, and contributions to media)

NB: 'Death education' should not be interpreted to mean information about the agency's services. The content of death education is directed specifically at changing attitudes toward death, dying and loss and/or addressing ignorance in these areas.
At least two of the above.

3   Demonstrated evidence of Education in Social Approaches to Care for:

    a   Staff (including Volunteers) [in-service education and higher education]
    b   Caregivers [in-service]
    c   Community (talks, publications, and contributions to media)

NB: 'Social education' means teaching people to view the experience of living with a life-threatening illness in terms of social alterations, eg, work, church, friendships, sexual relations. Other issues of importance may be topics such as stigma and discrimination, unexpected popularity, living with loss, or communication and support difficulties.
At least two of the above

4   Demonstrated evidence of non-clinical partnerships:
With the aim of understanding prevention, harm-minimisation, early intervention, community development, participatory health care, health ecology, and the Ottawa Charter.

    a   Membership of Health Promotion/Public Health Associations
    b   Regular meetings with Community Health Agencies
    c   Annual attendance at a public health conference by some staff/volunteers Schools

At least (a) and one other activity

5   Education Resource Material
NB: The resource collection should contain client AND professional material. In this way the reading material should cater for patient, family and staff needs.

    a   Death Education Literature/audio-visuals. These might include books and articles of grief and loss and also near-death experiences and visions, spiritual issues in death and dying, world culture and customs in death and dying, sociology of death and dying, first person accounts of living with life-threatening illness and caring for those people.
    b   Complimentary Therapy Literature/audiovisuals. These might include, for example, books on Reiki, therapeutic touch, massage, aromatherapy, and meditation. These topics are relevant for symptom control and quality of experience.
    c   Health Promotion Literature/audiovisuals. Much of this literature is for staff development. These might include literature on health promoting palliative care, health promoting environments, health education, sexual health, and community development.
    d   Spirituality Literature/audiovisuals. These might include literature about a range of reflective and meditative (anecdotes, quotations, poems, etc) literature for clients; and for staff in spiritual and pastoral care in palliative care settings.

A library containing these items should be in evidence. These might include books and copies and collections of journal articles.

6   Social Research

a   Evidence of partnerships in research devoted to social issues in palliative care
b   Staff reading groups or journal clubs devoted to social, cultural and spiritual research topics
c   Actual social research activities
d   Encouraging staff toward future education in welfare studies, public health, social sciences, humanities, or legal and political studies.

7   Policy
Evidence of regular submissions to:

a   Local Members (MPs)
b   Government committees of inquiry
c   Department Of Human Services
d   Local councils
e   Peak bodies (eg: PCV)

These submissions should describe agency activities, staff and client needs

8   Staffing Profile

a   Employment of socially trained professionals, especially social workers and pastoral care workers
b   Access to a health promotion and/or health educator worker
c   A staff profile that resembles the cultural and social profile of the community in which it serves

The annual report should be able to identify what proportion of funding was devoted to these staff issues, services, and consultancies.

9   Evidence of Health Promoting Settings

a   Minimisation of impact of clinical settings
b   Environments that recognise and enhance individual identity
c   Environments that provide opportunities for community access and participation
d   Environments that provide genuine opportunities for health improvements (relief of distress – emotional, physical, social and spiritual, physical mobility, sense of wellbeing, etc.)

10 Demonstrated Community Development Program

    a   Provides regular partnered and cooperative activities
    b   With local government
    c   With local media
    d   With local schools, workplaces and churches
    e   With local community sporting, service and political groups
    f   Raising awareness about death, dying, loss and caring

These guidelines are meant to be read in conjunction with the theory and philosophy of *Health Promoting Palliative Care* (Kellehear 1999) available from Oxford University Press Australia.
© Palliative Care Unit, La Trobe University Melbourne, 2003

Copies of this document are available from: La Trobe University Palliative Care Unit, La Trobe University (City Campus) 215 Franklin Street Melbourne, Victoria 3000

    All comments, criticism and additions are most welcome.
Email: palled@latrobe.edu.au
Tel: (03) 9285 5259
Fax: (03) 9285 5111
Web: www.latrobe.edu.au/publichealth

Appendix 4

An action plan for the initiation of a palliative care in the service in the community

The Neighbourhood Network in Palliative Care, Kerala

Step I

Sensitisation: Get those who are likely to be interested to an awareness meeting/ discussion. Make sure that all the groups/organisations involved in social/health care activities in the region are invited. Explain the issue of incurably ill/bed ridden patients in the region. Discuss possible way to help them. Register those who are willing to spend a couple of hours every week for such patients as volunteers.

Step II

Train those who are willing to get trained in basic nursing care and communication skills/emotional support. Get them to document the problems of bed ridden/incurably ill patients in their neighbourhood (Use a proper form like the community volunteers protocol). Discuss solutions in the group. Initiate a social support program. Start collecting money, manpower and other resources. Link with the nearest palliative care unit if one is available.

Step III

Get the services of a nurse. Encourage the nurse to get trained in palliative care. Initiate nurse led home care programs.

Step IV

Get help from a local doctor in medical issues. Encourage the doctor to get trained in palliative care.

Step V

Initiate Outpatient clinic/Inpatient services with the trained doctor and nurse.

Step VI

Continue with steps I and II.

Appendix 5

Model of Palliative Care, Lothian, Scotland

NHS Lothian

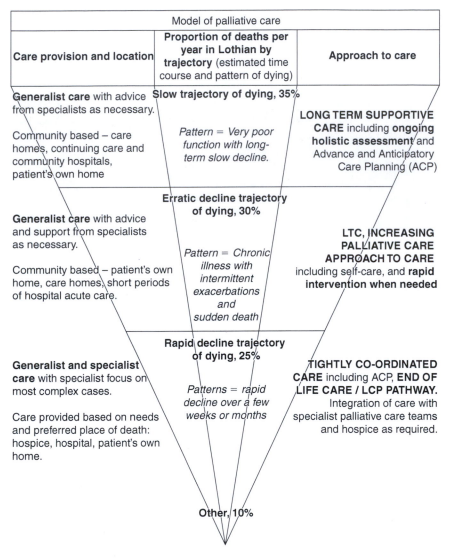

	Model of palliative care	
Care provision and location	**Proportion of deaths per year in Lothian by trajectory** (estimated time course and pattern of dying)	**Approach to care**
Generalist care with advice from specialists as necessary. Community based – care homes, continuing care and community hospitals, patient's own home	**Slow trajectory of dying, 35%** *Pattern = Very poor function with long-term slow decline.*	**LONG TERM SUPPORTIVE CARE** including **ongoing holistic assessment** and Advance and Anticipatory Care Planning (ACP)
Generalist care with advice and support from specialists as necessary. Community based – patient's own home, care homes, short periods of hospital acute care.	**Erratic decline trajectory of dying, 30%** *Pattern = Chronic illness with intermittent exacerbations and sudden death*	**LTC, INCREASING PALLIATIVE CARE APPROACH TO CARE** including self-care, and **rapid intervention when needed**
Generalist and specialist care with specialist focus on most complex cases. Care provided based on needs and preferred place of death: hospice, hospital, patient's own home.	**Rapid decline trajectory of dying, 25%** *Patterns = rapid decline over a few weeks or months*	**TIGHTLY CO-ORDINATED CARE** including ACP, **END OF LIFE CARE / LCP PATHWAY.** Integration of care with specialist palliative care teams and hospice as required.
	Other, 10%	

Figure A5.1 Model of palliative care (source: NHS Lothian (2010) *Living & Dying Well in Lothian – Lothian's Palliative Care Strategy 2010–2015*. www.nhslothian.scot.nhs.uk/ladwinlothian/).

Appendix 6

Survey questionnaire for HOME Hospice for Chapter 10

Home Hospice

Primary caregiver's details

Date: _____

1 Primary caregiver's name: _____ Age: _____ Sex: M ☐   F ☐
2 What is the primary caregiver's relationship to the patient: _____
3 What other activities and responsibilities does the primary caregiver have?
   Work for income ☐ Family to care for ☐ Other ☐
4 What are the religious beliefs of the primary caregiver? _____
5 What is the primary caregiver's state of health?
   Well ☐ Average ☐ Sick ☐
6 What are the main concerns of the primary caregiver? _____

Patient's details

7 Patient's name: _____ Patient's Age: ___ Sex: M ☐   F ☐
8 What illness does the patient have?
   Cancer ☐   HIVAIDS ☐   Other ☐
9 Who else is living in this home with the patient?

Table A

Name	Relationship	Age

10 What are the religious beliefs of the patient? _____
11 Is there any income coming into this patient's home? Yes ☐   No ☐
12 What activities and responsibilities does the patient have?
    Work for income ☐ Family to care for ☐ Other ☐
13 What are the main concerns of the patient? _____

HOME Hospice facilitator's details

14 HOME Hospice facilitator's name: _____   Sex: M ☐   F ☐
15 How long have you been involved supporting the primary caregiver as the home hospice facilitator? _____
16 How many family, friends and neighbours were supporting the primary caregiver? _____
17 *Table B*

What activity was done to support the primary caregiver by their family, friends and neighbours?	*Who did this activity to support the primary caregiver?*

18 As home hospice facilitator, what was the best thing you did to support this primary caregiver?_____
19 Do you believe that hh helped this family situation? Why? _____

Details of the patient's death

20 Date patient died:_____
21 How did the patient die?   Peacefully ☐   With difficulty ☐
    Comforted ☐   Someone with them ☐   Alone ☐   Fearful ☐
22 AS HOME Hospice facilitator, what was the best thing you did to support this primary caregiver when the loved one was dying or died?_____
    _____
23 Are there any orphans in this family?   Yes ☐   No ☐
24 Do you know what has happened to the orphans?
    Gone to orphanage ☐   Remained in the home ☐
    Moved away to live with family ☐   Not known ☐
    Taken in and cared for by neighbours and other village members ☐
25 As HOME Hospice Facilitator for this Primary Caregiver please can you tell us about any other COMMENTS, IDEAS or EXPERIENCES told to you by the dying loved one, Primary Caregiver and their community about HOME Hospice.

Index

Page numbers in *italics* denote tables, those in **bold** denote figures. Not all cited authors are listed in the index; readers requiring complete lists of cited works and authors should consult the reference lists at the end of each chapter.